To Maudie 12/5/17

With ?

+

~ cwo

The Power or Bailey, Bach and Verbeia Essences for Animals

Caroline Thomas

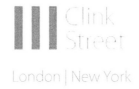

London | New York

Published by Clink Street Publishing 2017

Copyright © 2017

First edition.

ISBN:
978-1-911525-73-8 - paperback
978-1-911525-74-5 - ebook

www.emotionalhealing4animals.co.uk

'Owner of the Hoof and Paw Academy'

Dedicated to my two wonderful sons

Michael and Conor.

And my very supportive husband Jim

Contents

Foreword
By Rebecca Hunter

If you love the animals in your life, this book is for you!

Anyone who has a pet knows that they are sensitive and emotional beings. Simply providing food and warmth is not enough for their total well-being. We need to address their emotional needs as well. This is what flower essences are for.

I sometimes think of flower essences as little bottles filled with miracles. The speed with which they work can be quite astounding. I've seen animals make a complete turnaround almost instantly, and I've seen animals take several weeks to respond. But very rarely have I come across a case where there was no positive change in behaviour after taking essences.

In this book, Caroline will introduce you to the world of flower essences and help you to discover which ones can be used to help your animal through their own particular emotional difficulties.

I met Caroline in 2016 when she came up to Yorkshire to visit the home of the Bailey Flower Essences. She wanted to immerse herself in Arthur's work in order to better understand the essences. Her passion for her subject shines through in conversation and in her writing.

This book is easy to read and has full instructions on choosing flower essences and on the different ways that you can use them with your pet.

There is an amazing depth of knowledge here. It's all covered. Everything from the basic needs of your pet through to their emotional and spiritual make-up; how you can help them (and yourself) to find true happiness and contentment in life and full details of Bailey, Bach and Verbeia flower essence ranges.

Make no mistake, this book will give you great insight into the mind of your pet and give you the tools and knowledge to make a difference in their lives. It's an entertaining read and I found it hard to put down.

Well done Caroline – this book is a testament to your love of animals and your generosity of spirit.

Rebecca Hunter

Rebecca has worked with flower essences since the mid-1980s, largely under the wing of Arthur Bailey, creator of the Bailey Essences. She started the Bailey Essences business with Chris and Arthur in the early 1990s and has recently passed this work on to Jenny Howarth (creator of Verbeia essences).

About the Author

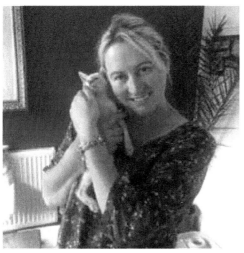

Caroline lives in Essex in the United Kingdom where she practises and teaches various holistic therapies. She specialises in Flower Essence Therapies for animals and has been very privileged to treat a large array of animals using flower essences. Caroline has worked with some very complex cases, which include a wide variety of animal species. To prepare for this book, she has treated over 80 animals across the globe. This has given her the evidence to show how beneficial Bailey, Bach and Verbeia essences can be. Some of the cases are included here to demonstrate the amazing properties that these essences have. Caroline has been given permission by Rebecca Hunter, the daughter of Arthur Bailey, to write this book. She has made lifelong friendships with the owners of the animals that she has worked with, and built strong professional relationships with vets. Often, Caroline has been completely in awe from the results as she sees both physical improvements as well as emotional advances.

Caroline has been using flower essences with animals for over 14 years; working closely with the Facebook group Autism In Dogs, offering flower essences advice. She specialises in helping rescue animals and in past years worked very closely with the Remus Horse

Sanctuary. She considers them to be one of the most forward-thinking sanctuaries in the UK in terms of their holistic care. Caroline has learnt what works and what does not. She is a qualified Animal and Human Bach Flower Practitioner, EFT Practitioner, qualified Animal Aroma therapist and Animal Reiki Master and teacher. She is very passionate about sharing her knowledge, so is a guest writer for three holistic animal websites. Caroline has also created a range of holistic crystal collars for dogs and has proven that when made with the correct holistic care, they can make a huge difference to the animal wearing them.

She has created an online academy where she can teach animal therapies to students all over the world. She believes that anyone can learn when nurtured and praised if given a variety of tools to do so. She uses supportive tools such as words, visuals, audio and art.

Caroline has been happily married for over 25 years and has two amazing sons. Her other passions are her two dogs, Tara and Lenny, and her two cats, Reuben and Matilda.

Introduction

I have been working with flower essences for many years, teaching numerous students how to use flower essences with animals. This book was initially written to reflect the powers of the Bailey essences but in the five years it has taken me to write this book, I found out that Arthur Bailey had developed a Bach Flower Essences range and Jenny Howarth of the Bailey Essences had developed her own Verbeia range, which she had created on the Ilkley Moors, Verbeia being the Celtic-Roman goddess of Wharfdale. Ilkley is the location of the Bailey Essence headquarters, where essences have been made for over 50 years.

The most important thing for me is to make the Bailey, Bach and Verbeia Essences interesting and easy to understand, as I appreciate that it can often be very overwhelming in the beginning. It is important to teach from experience and to share what I have learnt from the animals, always remembering that they know best.

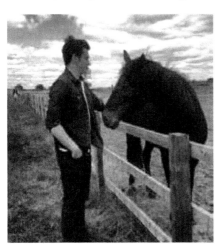

Left to their own devices in the wild, animals have for thousands of years been able to self-medicate with herbs, choosing them for their individual healing properties. Animals have long been able to connect with the energy from surrounding nature. With the dew on the petals of certain flowers, animals knew instinctively what the flower contained and would eat those petals. This would offer them the uplifting emotional property they were seeking. Animals were far more aware of the energy of flowers, long before the discovery of the powerful energies of plants by man.

It goes without saying that for the Bailey, Bach and Verbeia Essences to work on animals, they too must have emotional feelings. This is a topic that could fill another book; but it is often misunderstood or overlooked that they feel just as deeply as humans. They feel depressed, they grieve, they get stressed in the same way that we do. You may not see the tears, but do not be mistaken, they are sentient emotional beings just like us.

Unfortunately, our animals are living in the processed material world that we have provided, and they often find it difficult to be the animal they were intended to be.

This book will help you to understand how your animal is truly feeling. You will need to put yourself in their paws, to see them emotionally from their point of view. Their behaviour will usually reflect anything stressful going on in their lives. It is up to you to be a detective to find out what is causing their stress, and to heal their problems with the power of the Bailey, Bach and Verbeia Essences.

Understanding how our pets tick is key to finding the correct essence to help them. Open your mind to the Bailey, Bach and Verbeia Essences and see the magic unfold.

The History of Bailey Flowers Essences

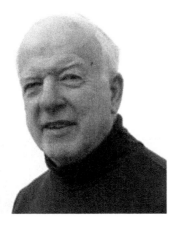

Who was Arthur Bailey? I got to know of Arthur about six years ago, through his amazing book about Dowsing for Health. In the work that I do, I often read books to help me with my own holistic learning. There was something very different about Arthur, and I was very drawn to him as a person. I loved his scientific mind and the way he could easily explain things in terms that made it easy for me to understand. In some ways, we both approached things in a similar way, as in my day job I am a Registered Pharmacy Technician. There was a strong connection from the moment I started to read his book.

In the 1960s Arthur become ill after contracting the Asian flu. It left him completely debilitated and he was eventually diagnosed with M.E. At that time, there was little known about this condition; but it left Arthur lacking energy, he felt exhausted all the time. As he was often confined to his bed, it was during this time that he read lots of books on varying subjects, on topics that he would not have been interested in before. One of the books he read was a book on dowsing. He was totally fascinated with this topic, and this was the start of a long journey; one which would change his life forever. It opened him up to a whole new subject matter and brought along many possibilities and new opportunities. Arthur had a curious mind and would spend hours around his home, dowsing for pipes, water, metal etc. He wanted to know how it worked and why it worked, what the potential benefits were and ultimately how it could help him with his own illness. He read book after book as he had an insatiable thirst for knowledge. He was a grounded individual and he would not take things at face value. His scientific mind would always question why and how things should be. It was then that he discovered the Bach Flower Essences which helped him with his illness. Dowsing offered him a tool to find a combination of flower essences for his clients. It allowed him to connect to their soul and to truly understand what was going on. He realised that dowsing could offer so many other opportunities and in his book, he explored many interesting ideas.

Arthur was fascinated by flowers at a young age and found a mentor in George Ringer, who was the husband of his grandmother's housekeeper in Cumbria, England. Arthur would have many adventures with George, roaming the woods and countryside.

It was early on in his dowsing career that Arthur began finding flower essences. In 1967, he found the first six in his garden using dowsing. This was the beginning of a wonderful discovery of the workings of dowsing and flower essences. He would use his intuition to find the flowers and would often sit with them, listening to what they had to say. The more he worked with flowers the more his intuition grew, allowing him to understand what each flower was for.

I have never met Arthur, but from the first moment I read his book I was fascinated. For me it was an eye-opening experience as his scientific approach made total sense. From that instant, I knew I had to write a book about how the essences work with animals.

Arthur died in 2008 leaving Chris, his loving wife and companion. Chris and her daughter Rebecca continue his work in the same manner as he did.

The ways that the Bailey Flower Essences are made are very interesting as they often contain not only the flower, but also other parts of the plant in some cases. This is very insightful and is what gives these essences their extra special properties. For some reason, animals truly resonate with these essences, perhaps due to their animalistic nature that allows them to connect on a deeper level. They are uncomplicated and are made with the purest intention. Animals like things that are not complicated; they specifically like energies that are not polluted by an 'ego'.

Arthur could make these essences so that only the flowers speak for themselves. In life, we are often leading our animals: telling them what to eat, where to sleep, who to be friends with. Yet 'being' with your animal is so much more powerful, as you allow your animal to take control of their own healing. Take the time to just sit with your animal, with no expectations, and you will be amazed at how stimulating that is for you both. We are always rushing from here to there, but when you stop and take the time to smell the flowers, it will open an unspoken understanding between you and your pet.

Dog Behaviour

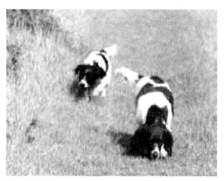

Dogs make a family; they are loving, caring, loyal and consider themselves in an instant to be at the centre of the family. They can be your best confidant, your exercise buddy and will never judge for what you might say or how fat you may be. They make a house feel like a home, and when they are not there it feels empty. They have filled my life with new adventures, often joyful, sometimes challenging, but always rewarding.

For example, one time my Tara got into my two bins, and when I came downstairs the kitchen floor was horrendous. She chewed through my brand new mobile phone and expensive curtains, and ate my son's cricket gloves the day before he left for a cricket tour. My other dog, Megan, had chewed through a first edition of a limited book and swallowed my diamond earrings.

In difficult moments like this it is easy to get angry and frustrated. But you should always remember the loyalty of a pet; soon after an operation Megan stayed by my side for weeks, just willing me to get well.

A dog is a friend, a companion that will love you unconditionally and see the true spirit of your heart. They ask for nothing, only to share in your life.

- Dog behaviour in part is due to the close and far-reaching relationship that dogs have with humans. This also means that dogs have a unique understanding of our behaviour. Dogs are a social species, so they need companionship from other dogs. In single-dog-only homes, they transfer their need for companionship to people or other animals in the household. They cannot be left alone for long periods of time as they crave companionship. If left on their own for long periods, it can lead to 'separation anxiety' which may lead to them barking, howling, digging or chewing.

- How dogs became domesticated is unclear but it is believed that dogs evolved from wolves. They communicate in a very similar way to that of wolves: scent marking, submission, smelling each other and barking or howling.
- Dogs are pack animals, with a hierarchy based on pack order, and they will fill a void if there is no obvious 'top dog'. (This hierarchy behaviour is being questioned by scientists but it has always made sense to me.) Humans take on this role; but if they lead weakly, it causes problems if the dog is unsure of the pack order. Dogs like structure and fair discipline, and like to play too. In fact, they love to play.
- Dogs are territorial animals and will defend that territory if threatened.
- Dogs have a highly advanced olfactory system which is a thousand times more sensitive than that of the human nose.
- Dogs need to be socialised from a young age, to other dogs, people and experiences. Or they may be fearful, which could lead to fearful aggression.
- Dogs need to be exercised on a regular basis; they need to let off steam, to experience different smells, and to have the chance to meet other dogs.
- It is important to recognise that different breeds are bred for different purposes. Therefore, they may need altered types of exercise and stimulation to meet their individual needs.
- Dogs like a varied diet and can eat both meat and plants. If left to their own devices, they would scavenge almost anything; it is a natural trait that means they have been known to eat out of bins, if given the chance.
- Dogs peak at dusk and dawn, so at these times they may be more excitable, barking, jumping or chewing.
- Dogs like to be stimulated and to play games that will stretch their imagination. This is very important with dogs that live on their own.

Cat Behaviour

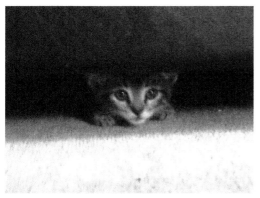

Cats have evolved from the African wild cat. If you have the time, Google this cat and you will see that it looks just like your local moggy. They were revered by the Egyptians, who worshipped them. Foreign travellers saw them as sacred, and took them back to their homeland. It was here that they adapted to every situation they met, adapting with the cold, the food and environment, and have since managed to reach almost every single part of the earth. They are the 'people's pet'. There's no need to walk them, no need to get home at an exact time to feed the cat. They can use a litter tray so do not need to be let out. On the surface, they are the 'purrfect' animal to have for a busy lifestyle. They do not have the same high maintenance demands as that of a dog.

We must, however, remember that we are living with a wild animal, which may have evolved socially into our cuddly beloved pet. They still need us to respect their animal instincts. We need to understand that cats are 'unique'. They are 'predators' who hunt the birds and the mice in our local neighbourhood. They are also the 'prey' of the neighbourhood however, always worried by the dog lurking behind the corner waiting to pounce. Cats have this unique title, which helps us to understand where they are coming from: to see how they operate, and how they see and understand the world.

- Cats were initially domesticated in Cyprus around 9500 years ago, long before their adulation by Egypt.
- Kittens taken away from their mother too soon may be fearful. They have not learnt how to be a cat, so can find the world we live in very scary. They like to hide and don't like to be confronted with new situations. In reality, the early weeks are when they would be learning from their mum and siblings the language that is 'cat'.
- Cats 'literally' see their world through smell and have highly sensitive noses. They are always marking new things with their scent as it makes them feel secure. Scent marking includes us. Changes in their environment can be very stressful for them. Movement of furniture, new kitchen, new house extension, new cat, new baby etc. can cause them massive amounts of stress. When their environment is compromised, they will spray/ damage furniture and even pluck out their own hair.
- Cats are territorial and tomcats will defend their territories from other invading tomcats. Always best to neuter them.
- Cats like a bolt hole to hide in. Usually high up, where they can groom and sleep.
- Indoor cats need lots of stimulating of their senses.
- In the wild, cats are social and would form a social group, which is not unlike a pride of lions. Having too many cats can cause unnecessary stress.
- Cats don't like their food bowl to be left by their litter tray. Eating and defecating is a definite 'no'.
- Cats are meat eaters with a capital 'M'. No such thing as a vegetarian cat, I am afraid.

Horse Behaviour

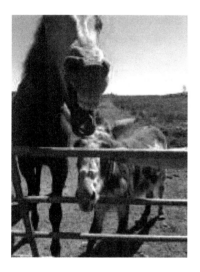

Out of all the animals I've worked with, I have a natural fascination with horses as to how they are treated and perceived by humans. Stress in horses has become a huge problem; I often get e-mails saying my horse is biting, my horse has terrible skin problems, my horse is aggressive. When I strip it all apart the answer is often quite simple. The owner doesn't understand what their horse is trying to say. How can it be right for a horse to be stabled for up to 18 hours a day and there not be retaliation such as biting or weaving? How can it be right for a horse to have more owners than a car has, and there not be a consequence of aggression, depression or skin problems? I have only met one horse who only had one owner. I am not saying that this is bad, I am just saying that this is a fact of life. Trying to fix Daisy 10 years down the line after she has had four previous homes is not always easy, but it is possible. With Bailey, Bach and Verbeia Essences there is no such word as impossible, as everything is always possible.

- Horses are prey animals and have a highly-developed flight and fight response. Deep down they still think there may be lions and tigers out there ready to pounce. We know that is not true; but try telling a horse that after millions of years of evolution.
- Horses were domesticated thousands of years ago, for a multitude of reasons from horse racing to pulling carts.

- Horses have evolved to live in herds, so that there are more eyes to see predators. They have a herd hierarchy structure, which helps to reduce aggression and yet at the same time increases unity. The pecking order is usually a linear system but who is in charge can have several factors, which will be dependent on an individual's need for a specific resource at a given time. They are social and like to hang out with the same friends, but the herd dynamics can change at any time depending on the reaction to a resource by a herd member.
- Horses form pair bonds, which mean they like to hang out with their best friend, literally all the time. These bonds can last for their entire lifetime. However, it has been known for horses to pair up with sheep, goats, etc. if they are deprived of mixing with other horses.
- Horses can sleep both standing up and lying down but lying down can make them more vulnerable to predators.
- Horses communicate to each other via smell, visual signals, grooming and, of course, vocalisations.
- Horses have a strong grazing instinct and love browsing for herbs, shrubs, twigs and leaves. They walk and graze at the same time.

Brambell's Five Freedoms

For nearly all animals that have human caretakers, virtually everything in their lives is at their owner's mercy and out of the animal's control; what happens then is that the owner's predominant emotions and responses become the guidance mechanism for the animal as to when they need to experience any of the Five Freedoms below. The Brambell Report stated, 'An animal should at least have sufficient freedom of movement to be able without difficulty, to turn round, groom itself, get up, lie down and stretch its limbs'. Also, what happens when the owner is unable to meet the freedoms? Is it then animal cruelty? The Five Freedoms are used as the basis to audit the basic needs of an animal by organisations such as veterinarians and the RSPCA.

In 1965, Professor Roger Brambell was asked to investigate how animals are farmed intensively. This was partly due to a book written by Ruth Harrison called Animal Machines which exposed the cruel reality of intensive farming. Brambell's investigation was the most comprehensive effort to define the basic needs of animals. Because of his investigation, Brambell made recommendations on how farm animals should be kept, called 'The Five Freedoms'; although initially for farm animals, they can apply to all animals including cats, dogs and horses. They can help us assess how well we are meeting our animal's needs and therefore their welfare. These simple rules can ensure that your animal is living as happily as they possibly can.

1. Freedom from thirst, hunger and malnutrition

- Does your animal have access to fresh water?
- Does your animal have a wholesome diet that is natural to their species? Remember it is us who chooses the time our animal eats and what they eat. Have we taken their free choice away?

- Do not overfeed your animal. In the wild, animals would only choose to eat what they need and what is good for them. You would never find an overweight animal in the wild!

2. Freedom from discomfort due to the environment

- Does your animal have an appropriate shelter and environment, which provides protection from temperature and weather extremes? Consider it from an animal's point of view. If whilst at work you have left the heating on, and your animal gets too hot, does it have the freedom to move somewhere cooler?
- Does your animal have a comfortable resting place of its own where it can feel safe and secure? – It is especially important for older dogs/cats and puppies/kittens to have a quiet safe area in an environment free from things that could cause harm.

3. Freedom from pain, injury or disease

- If your animal is unwell, it is important that they receive a rapid diagnosis by a qualified veterinarian. In the wild, animals would seek out healing herbs to help heal any ailments. Animals living in our homes are 100% reliant on us to seek out the care they need.
- Does your animal see a veterinarian on an annual basis? Prevention is the key to keeping your animal well.

4. Freedom to express normal behaviours for the species

- In the wild, horses would live in herds, dogs would live in packs. Does your animal have adequate opportunity to meet and interact with others of their own species? Dogs and cats are both social animals; although we think we can speak dog or cat and think we know what they are saying and need, dogs and cats on their own would truly benefit from meeting animals of their own kind. Many people think of cats as loners, but this is not true. They too enjoy company.
- Is your horse allowed to live with their pair bond/live in an established herd? A horse left on his own would be extremely stressed, as horses are prey animals. In the wild, they would always be in a herd.

- Does your dog get enough exercise? A pet that does not get enough exercise can become bored and frustrated. This could lead to them acting out behaviours which you may find undesirable.
- Your pet needs mental stimulation. This can be provided with a range of stimulating toys that you can use to play with them.

5. Freedom from fear and distress

- What can cause your animal fear and distress? Puppies and kittens taken away from their mothers too young can become fearful and distressed as they have not had time to learn from their mother and siblings the skills to be a confident young animal.
- To prevent an adult pet from being unsure of himself and fearful, it is essential that he has been socialised to as many new experiences as possible during the critical socialisation period.
- Protect your pet by avoiding stressful situations.
- Understand what is causing the stress and try to prevent it from happening. For example, your dog may be getting stressed by being left at home while you work. It is possible to work with a professional animal behaviourist as to how you can prevent this from happening.

Animal Welfare Law in the UK 2006

The Animal Welfare Act, which came into force in England and Wales in 2007, replaced the Protection of Animals Act, first passed in 1911. The Act was the first review of pet law in 94 years, introducing a welfare offence for the first time. This places a 'duty of care' onto pet owners to provide for the animal's basic needs, such as adequate food and water, veterinary treatment and an appropriate environment in which to live. The 1911 act only enforced a duty of care for farm animals. However, this newer bill does not include farm animals, as the government have given assurances that farm animals already have a high standard of care. Laboratory animal welfare and animals used for horse or greyhound racing are not included in the bill.

The Animal Welfare Act has given more powers to the RSPCA to intervene if they suspect a pet is being neglected and tougher penalties for an offence under Section Four. This section covers unnecessary suffering such as docking tails, poisoning and fighting. Those cases are liable on summary conviction to imprisonment for up to 51 weeks and fines of up to £20,000. They can also result in lifetime ban on some owners keeping any pets.

Tail docking for cosmetic reasons is banned, the exception being for working dogs such as those in the police and armed forces. Castrating, spaying and ear tagging are not illegal.

Similarly, the Animal Health and Welfare (Scotland) Act came into force in October 2006. It aimed to make the law more robust. The Act makes it an offence to 'fail to take reasonable steps to ensure the welfare of a protected animal' or to cause a protected animal unnecessary suffering.

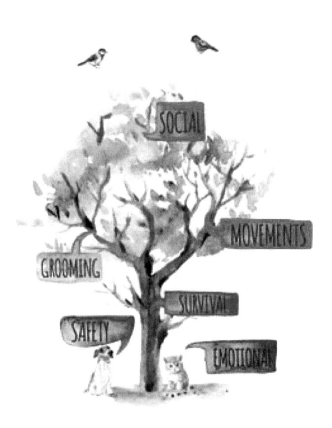

The Hoof and Paw Tree of needs

This is how I teach to my students in my Hoof and Paw Academy: I put the emotional needs first. It may not be the normal conventional theory but it has worked well for me over the last 14 years.

For animals to feel safe and relaxed, they need to have certain needs met and preferably in the order listed above. At the root of the tree, you have the emotional needs. A tree with strong roots will be able to withstand anything that blows their way. Meeting the emotional needs of your animal is key to keeping your animal well balanced and safe. This is the root and pathway to all your animal's happiness. If an animal is fearful or grief-stricken, they are going to care little about their survival and the need to find food. They will, however, need to urinate/defecate, drink and sleep. But this will be very difficult if their emotional and safety needs are not met first. An animal that is stressed will spend most of its time living on its nerves, pacing or may even have shut down completely. I have worked with horses that have lived in the most appalling conditions with little food or water. Once given the security of a loving home, it is then that their whole system shuts down. It is almost as if they have been hanging on until their safety needs are met so then they can die in peace. Would this end have been different if they had been treated with essences before they found their safety?

When we move on to the second need of our animal, which is safety, many would have thought it to have been the first; therefore it is so interesting to understand the Hoof and Paw Tree of needs when working with the Bailey, Bach and Verbeia Essences. The essences support an animal who is fearful, while they learn to cope with their fears in any of the situations that are making them frightened. When you look at a tree you can see that the roots need to be the strongest and grow widest, so that they can support the rest of the tree of behaviours.

When an animal feels happy, safe and secure, they will be able to successfully groom, move and can become social with other animals and humans.

If you had put social, movement and grooming as the most important behaviours, then you would have an upside down tree. This would of course be very unstable, causing the tree to topple over and to crash to the ground. Then of course you would have a dead tree! Making sure that our animals' emotional needs are met and that they are the foundation of an animal's happiness is the magic concrete underpinning your animal's wellbeing.

You must remember that our animals are living in a society that has changed considerably over the last 50 years. It has become almost unrecognisable to both animals and humans. The food is now processed, the cities are polluted and the green fields destroyed by building new homes. Understandably animals are displaying more and more mental health issues because we have forgotten the basics of how to look after them and how to support their daily needs.

Bailey, Bach and Verbeia Essences are the perfect 'safe' therapy to support the myriad of behaviours that our animals are displaying. All the essences have a beautifully untouched energy that is pure and very honest. This is because they are made by hand and not in an automated busy factory. How an essence is made is extremely important in how it performs. You will be able to tackle any emotional problem as there is a huge selection of essences to choose from. This will help you to finely tune your selection of essences for your animal. It will make you re-access what is really going on emotionally for your animal and what is at the root of the problem. When did it start and what was the cause of this new behaviour?

Having a tree that is well nourished by the rain feeding its roots and the sunlight shining on the leaves is the same as an animal being fed correctly with the correct diet and being socialised to as many different experiences as possible from a young age. A healthy tree will weather all that comes its way and will stand strong in the hardest storm. It will offer protection to the birds and shelter the rabbits. For animals to be healthy and happy they need to be given the correct tools to grow emotionally and physically. When they do not receive the correct input, it is here that the Bailey, Bach and Verbeia Essences can be very beneficial.

How the Bailey Flower Essences are Made

This is where the magic happens, when the energy of the flower is transferred to water. It is a transfer of love and one of perfect symmetry. The delicate flower energy is then preserved in the water by using a preservative.

As Dr Bach did nearly 100 years ago, Bailey Flower Essences are made up mainly by using the sun method. (This is when the petals of the flower are placed in a bowl of water and left outside for a few hours on a sunny day.) Dr Bach did not want a shadow cast over the bowl with the flower head in and that was his preference. Arthur Bailey, however, was very clear that it is the intention with which an essence is made that counts the most, and not that the bowl was in a shadow. The only thing that he was careful about was making sure that the cats didn't drink the water! But otherwise, all the essences are made with care and reverence – but not undue reverence. It was Arthur's firm belief that everything is ordinary, or everything is extraordinary. It is the intention of the person making the essence that counts. The Bailey Essences team will not make any essences if they are feeling out of sorts. Also, they do not worry about clouds. Obviously the sun would be better but a sunny/cloudy day is fine. On cloudier days, it simply takes a little longer for the essence to be ready. The person making the essence has a great deal of input into the final essence. So it doesn't matter if their shadow falls across the essence as it is being made, since that person is already the one who has picked the flowers and made the essence. Arthur believed that we are all one with nature and that everything is connected.

What happens next is the beautiful handover of energy from the flower to the water. The simplest things often have the most powerful results. Dr Bach learnt very early in his discovery of flower essences that alcohol is the best preservative, so Bailey, like Bach, use alcohol to preserve their essences. They choose to use vodka, whereas Dr Bach preferred brandy.

Some of the Bailey flowers are not cut and are made by pouring water over the flower. This water is then collected to make up the essence. Each flower is treated individually on its own merit. For example, the Cymbidium Orchid is made by using the energy of the moon instead of the sun. I love that they choose to use different methods of extraction of the flower energy, which is based on the individual plant. Each method is listed with each of the descriptions of extraction on the following pages. It should be noted that one method does not fit all plants. I like the spiritual thought process for each plant as to how they were going to be used. It's a very forward-thinking process, which is why their energy is so special. The Bailey essences are known as a new generation of flower essences, and they work to help the mind, body and spirit of your animal.

Originally the essences were made up with the same dilution as the Bach Flower Essences. What makes the Bailey essences unique is that they are made in two stages. This gives the essences a greater potency. The first dilution from the 'mother' tincture is termed the 'daughter' tincture. This is tapped three or four times with the base of the thumb. This is the life force energy of the flower energy. The second stage of dilutions is the finished stock bottle.

The essences relate to the emotions of your animal and not to the actual disease. They will not fix the broken leg but what they will do is to help your animal to deal with the feelings surrounding the broken leg. As with people, animals will all behave differently even though the condition is the same. Some will be brave, some fearful, some uncontrollably stressed. Yet they will all have a broken leg that is broken in the exact same place, and how they heal will be dependent on how they feel. The Bailey Essences will alleviate the fear or stress and support the brave animal who shows no worry. They will allow healing to happen at the deepest level as it will be unhindered by any emotional baggage that is carried. The mind and the body are not separate entities and need to be seen as one. How one is treated will affect the other, so it is important to see them as a whole and this is why an animal living on their nerves will find it difficult to heal fully as their mind will not be relaxed, so their body will not be able to relax so their healing will be compromised.

The Bailey Essences are a catalyst for change for your animal to live in the 'now' and not stay in the past or yearn for the future. They want your animal to be present, they want you to be present with your animal. When taken along with giving the essences to your animal, they will allow a deeper bond to develop as you will both be in the 'now' space.

How the Bach Flower Essences are Made

Bach Flower Essences are made in the exact same way as Dr Bach intended. For me this shows the huge respect that Arthur had for Edward Bach's work, as the Bailey Essences are created in a very different way. The Bach Centre uses two methods to create its essences. Method one is the sun method. The delicate flower heads are floated in pure water for three hours in direct sunlight. The second method is used with woodier plants and those that bloom when the sun is weak. It is called the boiling method and involves boiling the flowering part of the plant for half an hour in pure water.

In both methods, there is a handover of energy from the flowers to the water. The energised water is mixed with an equal quantity of brandy. This mixture is called the 'mother tincture'. To make up a stock bottle, two drops of the mother tincture are added to 30ml of brandy.

How the Verbeia Essences are Made

The Verbeia Essences were created by Jenny Howarth, who is part owner of the Bailey Essences. Ilkley Moor has long been associated with healing powers and this is where Jenny found her inspiration for her Verbeia range. Jenny is a therapist and homeopath and the essences are made from moorland plants and the energy of the Wharfe Valley. Jenny was inspired to start her own range of flower essences around seven years ago, and has seven flower essences in her range.

The way that Jenny creates her essences is very different to that of Arthur Bailey or Dr Edward Bach. Jenny makes them from the growing plant. (This is ingenious as the plant will carry on living, after the procedure, until it is the time to naturally fade away.) She uses a peg and bamboo twigs to bend the plant down into the water. The Fylfot essence is made by carefully placing the essence bowl on one of the ancient carved stones of Ilkley Moor.

The name Verbeia comes from the name of a Celtic-Roman goddess who has a stone bearing her image inside the All Saints Parish Church in Ilkley. It is believed that she was worshipped by the Roman troops when they occupied Ilkley. There are many local stories of Verbeia's appearing in the Wharfe Valley.

The Verbeia Moorland essences have been made with honesty and care on Ilkley Moor. They have been carefully trialled by many, and the benefits experienced have been drawn together.

Getting to Know the Bailey Essences

Algerian Iris *(Iris Unguicularis)*

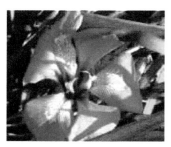

This essence makes us less susceptible to getting sexually involved in relationships that are inherently flawed.

Animals are born with an innate behaviour to protect their species. If left to their own devices, they would revert back to their survival structure. This flower allows a healthier view of sex. This flower essence would be excellent for dogs who have an obsession with their private parts, with the tendency to show you up while you are hosting guests.

It is made with the sun method using only the flowers.

Almond *(Prunus Dulcis)*

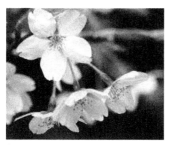

This essence is the supportive inner teacher, the guide. Forms links with our soul and encourages intuition.

This powerful essence will help animals to evolve from past behaviours that are serving no benefit. It helps to shine a light on the path in front, so that new skills can be learnt. Fear-based aggression is often held on to by the animal, as it provides a good safety mechanism to keep animals and people at bay. This behaviour restricts the animal's freedom; by taking this essence, new behaviours can be learnt which better suit the animal's situation.

It is made with the sun method using only the flowers.

Amaryllis *(Hippeastrum 'Piquant')*

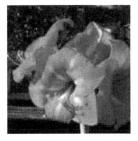

This essence gives the strength to speak from the heart with clarity and compassion. It will help animals to show how they truly feel. Animals speak to us from the heart every single day, and it is up to us to listen to them without judgement. This was the last essence that Arthur made and the first one that Rebecca made. A beautiful union for such a loving, supporting flower.

It is made by pouring water over the flowers until it feels complete.

Apricot Poppy *(Papaver Postii)*

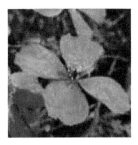

This essence brings beauty to barren areas as its beauty gently nurtures the animal to embrace change with love in their heart. It is a wonderful addition to other Bailey essences, as it whispers encouraging messages thereby enhancing their potential.

It is made with the sun method using only the flowers.

Arizona Fir *(Abies Koreana)*

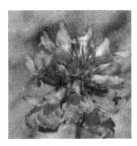

This essence helps us to celebrate life and existence as spiritually-based beings.

In life we need to have balance and this is especially important for animals. Clinging to woeful behaviours of doom and gloom or riding high on the energy of enjoyment. This essence allows the heart chakra to open, thereby allowing loving and acceptance of any flawed behaviour.

It is made with the alcohol method using the cones picked in summer.

Betony *(Stachys Officianlis)*

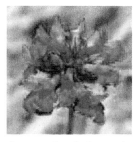

This essence is for fears that are hidden in the subconscious mind, including apparently irrational fears.

This flower is very favoured by animals and its properties make total sense as to the reason why. It is for 'fears' that are unrecognisable and undefinable, which to an animal are the greatest fears indeed. Something that cannot be quantified or recognised is often at the root of why animals are deeply unsettled and fearful. It gives animals permission to grow and develop, and much courage to explore the world they live in.

It is made with the sun method using only the flowers.

Bistort *(Polygonum Bistorta)*

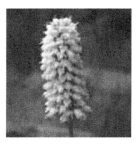

This essence provides loving support at times of major change in our lives.

This essence helps animals who are at a major change-point in their lives, which can be most relevant in cases where animals are abused. Their old ways of relating to the world are tested beyond their whole mental being. They are pushed to a point of deep mental turmoil. Bistort can help animals to look deep into their inner soul so they can awaken love and self-protection at times of major emotional upheaval. It offers a soothing comfort blanket of hope and optimism.

It is made using the alcohol method.

Black Locust (*Robinia Pseudoacacia*)

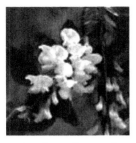

This essence is for protection against the negative influences of other people, including psychic attacks.

Definitely not black but its name is a good indicator of its properties. It is the essence of choice when animals feel vulnerable to the attacks, or undesired attentions, of other animals and people. Animals are very space-aware and some find it very difficult to cope when other animals or people invade their space, to a point that they will become aggressive. Dogs, due to extensive breeding and the fact that they are taken away from their mothers too young, are often unable to read the language of other dogs. Invading the space of another dog who is guarding their space can often cause a fight. As we know, animals are extremely psychic and sensitive to energies; this essence will also protect them from any energy that is unsettling to them.

It is made with the sun method using only the flowers.

Blackthorn (*Prunus spinosa*)

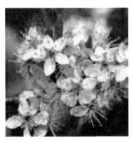

It is the remedy for the depths of despair – 'Valley of the Shadow of Death'.

Again the name of this flower is key to its properties. This blackness is for the ultimate state of despair, when there is no way out, trapped only by the darkness that is totally consuming. Animals at this point will often show this in their eyes. It is almost like they have checked out. They are emotionally dead and in fact death may be a blessing. Blackthorn mirrors these feelings with its sharp ominous thorns. Where there is dark, there is always the possibility of light and this light shines out from the beautiful white blossoms of hope. As light moves to dark, so will dark move to light, as this is the law of the universe. Blackthorn helps animals to accept their situation and brings hope to their very soul.

It is made with the sun method using only the flowers.

Bladder Senna *(Colutea x Media)*

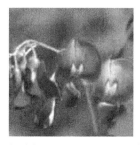

This essence is for escaping from feelings of guilt and being unworthy, brought about by judging ourselves far too harshly. It brings compassionate understanding of our past actions.

This beautiful flower supports animals to learn from past mistakes. Attachment of any sort can ultimately be unhealthy. Animals that hold on to past misdemeanours will often hinder their progress of moving forward to learn. Food aggression often stems from the lack of food and this is usually in the animal's formative years. This is carried with the animal into their adult life and even when they are given a healthy amount of food. The feelings of scarcity from when they were young are so overpowering that all common sense goes out the window. They are so emotionally linked to the feelings of scarcity that they will become food aggressive, and this can be dangerous to other animals and the owner. I gave this essence to a dog and as it worked its magic, it became clear that the dog never actually like the food he was given, yet he was so scared that he would never eat again; he was food aggressive for years. This essence allowed him to move forward and to be more choosy with his food and to enjoy his food.

It is made with the sun method using only the flowers.

Blue Pimpernel *(Anagallis arensis var. caerulea)*

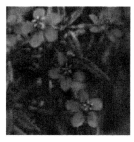

This essence is for rediscovering our spiritual nature whilst growing up in a superficial material world.

When you look at this flower, you can become dreamy and mesmerised in the depth of the colour of blue that this little flower reflects. It is a very spiritual flower and I believe with all my heart that animals have a spiritual soul. This flower offers insight and understanding of 'self-awareness'. It allows animals to be disentangled from their owner and yet, at the same time, be completely loyal to their owner.

It is made with the sun method using only the flowers.

Bluebell *(Hyacinthioides Non-Scripta)*

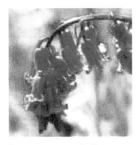

This essence is used where there has been depression, when one feels to be falling apart inside.

The typical Bluebell animal will have lost much of their confidence and this is due to a lack of support during their early years. Learning how to be an animal and the skills needed to hunt, to socialise, to communicate, are learnt in the formative years. This essence will help to restore self-esteem and will bring optimism where previously there has only been fear. 'Fear' is the biggest cause of so many emotional problems that are manifested in animals. Bluebell will unlock any hidden potential and help the animal to understand their distorted view of the world so they can grow in confidence to face their fears.

It is made with the sun method using only the flowers.

Bog Asphodel *(Narthecium Assifragum)*

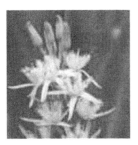

This essence is for the 'willing slave' – those who help others yet frequently ignore their own needs.

Loyalty in an animal is a trait that many owners look for. However, if this becomes all-consuming for the animal, this will be to the detriment of the animal. I am sure you have heard of dogs lying at their master's grave, never eating or drinking until they too are consumed by death. Bog Asphodel helps animals to look after their own needs and to view loyalty with a healthier attitude. It offers a brighter approach to life and may be a useful essence to consider in emotional problems such as separation anxiety in dogs. Dogs have a huge desire to serve their owner, which means being with their owner at every single moment; being separated causes them a huge amount of stress.

It is made with the sun method using only the flowers.

Bracken Alc *(Pteridium Aquilinum)*

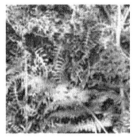

This essence is for where there has been a habitual playing of the 'child' role in life.

This essence is for animals who never truly grow up. This can be because they have not learnt the skills or because they have chosen to stay childlike. They will use their childlike behaviour to get their own way, which on the surface is submissive, yet it cloaks a feeling of deep resentment. Cats will often take on a juvenile role with their owners and show their under belly to be rubbed, yet in the blink of an eye they will swipe their owner with their sharp claws. The former sentence is an analogy, as animals have built-in behaviours to protect themselves. However, if this essence is chosen via dowsing, know in your heart that you have an animal who is very frustrated and is ready to let off steam, so beware.

It is made with the alcohol method using only the bracken fronds that have been used to make the Bracken Aquilinum with the sun method.

Bracken Aq. *(Pteridium Aquilinum)*

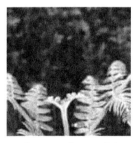

This essence is for when intuitive sensitivity was blocked in childhood, resulting in a fear of the intuitive side of one's nature.

This essence is very difficult to transcribe in terms of how it would help animals. The essence relates to the blocking of innate sensitivity in childhood. Animals who have an impaired understanding of the psychic are often in fear of the unknown. They will create all kinds of thoughts in their minds, which are not logical. They may appear unsettled and fearful. Bracken gently helps to unblock the intuitive mind so that both sides of the brain can come together to make sense of unnerving situations. Bracken will promote an increased feeling of harmony, so your animal will feel more at ease with situations that are unsettling.

It is made with the sun method using the new fronds of bracken as well as the old fronds from the previous year.

Butterbur *(Petasites Hydridus)*

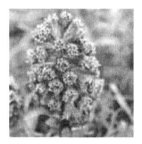

This essence is for blocked-off self-love, and not realising one's own inherent goodness.

This unusual flower is a powerful essence for aiding animals with low self-esteem. Animals who lack belief in themselves are often trapped in a world, where stepping out beyond their confidence can be very daunting for them. Their belief system in their worth can often stem from memories of being put down as a young animal by their owner. This may have been unintentional but the feelings from those words have stuck. They may have been told that they were not good enough, that they were 'naughty' and did not listen. Every word that we speak carries an energy and those with the hardest tone will be deeply ingrained in the very being of your animal. Butterbur will melt away those memories and allow your animal to let go of inferiority feelings and will help their self-esteem to blossom again.

It is made with the sun method, only using the flowers.

Buttercup *(Ranunculus Acris)*

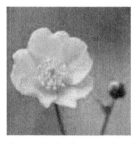

This essence is for those who find it difficult to let the 'sunshine' into their lives. It helps one to let go of embittered feelings.

This tiny yellow flower reminds me of a childhood memory, of holding the flower under my sister's chin and giggling to see if she liked butter. It oozes feelings of sunshine. Where there is darkness, let there be light. Often animals that have been abused will find it very difficult to trust again and sometimes impossible to trust again. This flower will allow them to understand that not all people are the same and whatever happened in the past will not necessarily happen again. It will allow your animal to have compassion and to see with their heart. Buttercup is the flower that will put your animal in touch with the flame of loving kindness that lies within everyone and everything.

It is made with the sun method using only the flowers.

Charlock *(Sinapis Aryensis)*

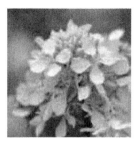

This essence is for the 'Peter Pans' of this world who cling to childhood states. They want to be liked and so often become habitual victims.

This flower will allow animals who find it difficult to grow up, the opportunity to be open to new challenges with the openness of a young animal. Moving from childhood to adulthood can often be a difficult passage. Charlock will offer clarity and awareness to situations and judgements which may otherwise be clouded by a childlike approach. When is an animal not grown up? Look for signs of over-exuberance and over-attachment.

It is made with the sun method using only the flowers.

Compact Rush *(Juncus Effusus)*

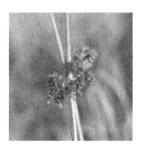

This essence is for lack of fulfilment; life seeming to pass one by. This essence assists new beginnings, new energies and new insights.

This is the essence for sadness, which is caused by a life that has passed by. When we try to understand this from an animal's point of view it is difficult to articulate because we do not know if our animals reflect on a life gone by. What we do know is that they do have memories of past abuse and can perhaps have suppressed anger for things that happened in their youth. They may feel resentful of the past wrongs, which leads to a sadness that things could have been different. Compact Rush is about starting afresh and will encourage your animal to see the present moment with new eyes and new insights.

It is made with the sun method using only the flowers.

This flower was originally misidentified. The correct Latin name is now listed, but the common name should really be Soft Rush.

Conifer Mazegill *(Gloeophyllum Sepiarium)*

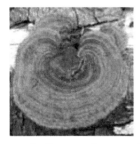

This essence is for sudden, irrevocable changes in our lives. It continually activates energies of positive change.

This essence is made from a beautiful bracket fungus that lives on dead conifer wood. It is stunningly beautiful and the first essence I have personally come across that is made from a fungus. It is a powerful essence for anything that is life-changing in your animal's life, which includes anything that is sudden or abrupt. Gosh! In an animal's life that could cover a multitude of events. Bereavement would be at the top of my list, along with change of owner, change of food, environment etc. When something has to die it is replaced by something new, just like the Conifer Mazegill which mirrors this exactly by replacing dead wood with new growth. This is a perfect example of the doctrine of signatures. With animals you have to think 'literally' so if anything happens that is sudden or abrupt, think of this essence.

It is made with the sun method using a piece of the fungus.

Cymbidium Orchid *(Cymbidium Hybridus)*

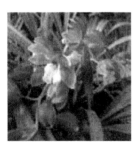

It relates to the hidden side of our nature, brings peace and harmony to the subconscious parts of our mind.

This is a lunar essence, made at the time of the full moon at the Bailey meditation room. By choosing to work with the moon energy an extra energy layer is added. This essence works with the Yin aspect of your animal, which is the dark side. When their feelings are repressed feelings of any kind, this essence will help to bring these feelings to the surface, Cymbidium brings insight and wisdom into your animal's intuition so that they can see that where there is Yin, there is always going to be Yang. This essence is about balance.

It is made in the light of the full moon, in lightly salted water using just the flowers.

Cyprus Rock Rose *(Fumana Arabica)*

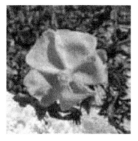

This essence is for deep terrors and fears that are difficult to expose and resolve.

Lack of socialisation is the biggest cause of fear in animals. It is crucial to socialise animals with as much stimuli as possible when they are young, otherwise you will end up with a very stressed and fearful animal. This essence is the perfect essence for the most extreme fear that your animal could experience. When your animal is shaking and trembling to their very core, that it stops them in their tracks, think of this essence. The shining sunlight of the Cyprus Rock Rose brings illumination to all the dark places that hold your animal in a state of fear or terror. This flower will help your animal to take stock of the present fearful situation, learn from it and then move forward.

It is made with the sun method using only the flowers.

Deep Red Peony *(Paeonia Lactiflora 'Suminoichi')*

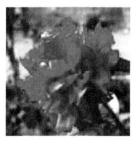

This essence reflects our spiritual life-blood, helping us to discover our true spiritual destiny. It encourages latent powers of energy and wisdom at a gentle pace.

This is a very powerful essence that will shine a light on a path that may otherwise lay undiscovered. It is useful for animals with behaviours like those of Asperger's, Attention Deficit Disorder and Hyperactivity Syndrome. Our animals are mirroring our human world at every level, hence the mirroring of these conditions. They are usually very highly intelligent animals who become disinterested very quickly and as a result are often disengaged from the world. This essence will allow your animal to grow up at their own pace.

It is made with the sun method using only the flowers.

Delphinium *(Delphinium Consolida)*

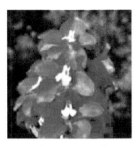

This flower will help your animal to widen their horizons. It will give them a bigger insight into problems and situations that they find difficult to encounter, encouraging your animal to go outside their comfort zone. When there is a perception of a situation being fearful, this essence will help them to bravely move forward and to step out of their fear zone. This essence catalyses the opening of our intuitive faculties.

It is made with the sun method using only the flowers.

Dog Rose *(Rosa Canina)*

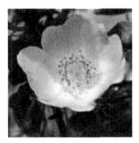

This essence is for loving comfort and support; it offers help along our path when life gets difficult. Dog Rose is a pretty pink flower that mirrors the properties of love and compassion – those of the 'heart protector' which is a fire element. This beautiful flower can help your animal when they need support and understanding as it comes from a place of love. When your animal has been deeply hurt such as in the loss of a companion, Dog Rose offers a warm comforting hug and will go even further to protect your animal from any negative influences. It will allow your animal to open up to you so your bond together will deepen.

It is made with the sun method using only the flowers.

Double Snowdrop *(Galanthus Nivalis 'Flore Plena')*

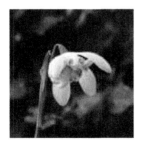

This essence is for when there are frozen attitudes and approaches to life. This essence brings openness; a lighter touch.

Double Snowdrop is for those animals who are stuck in the same learning patterns and need to have more flexibility in their lives. In the physical aspect, it can be used for animals who are frozen to the spot with fear. Animals like routine and will often cling on to old habits which now serve no purpose, only in the fact that they offer comfort. They need to understand that everything is constantly changing. This essence would suit animals who have not been socialised enough to their environment. Hence, they stay rooted to old behaviours, as they find it very uncomfortable to change. Double Snowdrop helps to break up the crusts of rigid attitudes that are keeping out joy and freedom, and to build trust and a sense of security through a period of transformation.

It is made with the sun method using only the flowers.

Dwarf Purple Vetch *(Vicia Villosa ssp. Eriocarpa)*

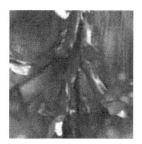

This essence is for deep-rooted, hidden patterns, usually originating in childhood and often resulting in sexual difficulties.

The Dwarf Purple Vetch comes from the mountains of Cyprus and grows in very rocky conditions on the mountains. It will allow your animal to let go of behaviours that were set when they were young. Especially those relating to sexual attitudes. Often these behaviours are deeply set. Understanding of the opposite sex is often blocked as the over whelming desire to understand it takes precedence, yet there is an underlining 'fear' of being misunderstood. It will offer your animal the key to the door of true personal and sexual freedom.

It is made with the sun method using only the flowers.

Early Purple Orchid *(Orchis Mascula)*

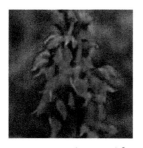

This essence is for unblocking the energy centres of the body and protecting any vulnerable spaces created.

The Early Purple Orchid helps to dissolve the blocks that are impeding your animal's progress. When the chakras and meridian system of your animal are blocked, it makes it difficult for them to communicate with you and other animals. If you think of a river flowing through the mountains, as time goes by boulders topple into the river.

Eventually the river becomes blocked and everything backs up behind the block and nothing can move past. Every emotion, every setback in your animal's life equally blocks their chakra and meridian system. Because these blocked areas distort your animal's main energy systems, they stop the flow of energy. This can and does affect their lives. Often your animal will remain stuck in the same behaviours of the past, as it is often easier to polish the bars of the bird cage instead of flying out through the open door.

It is made with the sun method using only the flowers.

Firethorn *(Pyrancantha Atalantioies)*

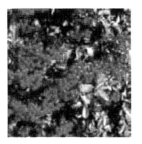

This essence is concerned with balancing up the 'fire' energy. This imbalance can be due to long-suppressed emotions.

Firethorn is the essence for helping your animal to balance their energies. Animals with unstable energies will often have suppressed emotions that will stay hidden until they finally lash out. After this outburst, if will often lead to panic with a need to retreat. Which can lead to an alternating energy of blowing hot and cold, making life very difficult for the animal's owner. Firethorn animals may be over-emotional in all that they do. They may be possessive of their toys, people or places. It is important for your animal to have a balanced energy, Firethorn will allow their energy to ebb and flow which will allow calmness to ensue. With the calmer energy, it is easier to see what the problem was.

It is made with the alcohol method using only the berries.

Flame Azalea *(Rhododendron Calendulaceum)*

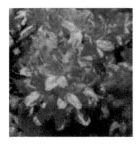

This essence helps us to regain our vital life force and sense of community after major changes in life.

The powerful Flame Azalea is a reminder that spring is here. The colour of the blossom mirrors the energy of renewal, of a powerful reawakening. It is as if the flower reminds the woods that a new time is dawning, a time for new visions and new horizons. The beautiful perfume reminds us that our life is to be freely shared with others in just the way that the azalea perfume is freely given for the delight of others.

This flower reminds your animal that the most natural thing is to be social. This essence would be particularly useful for animals who have difficulty integrating with other animals and humans.

The flower gives a message of renewing your power and energy. Whenever your animal faces an uncertain future it will help them to cope with what life is bringing to them; this is the essence of choice. It will help them to regain their vital life force and to cooperate lovingly with others, bringing with it a sense of loving purpose. Flame Azalea is particularly suitable for your animal when they have had a major irrevocable change in their life; bereavement, abuse or house move. Taken with Conifer Mazegill, it will help your animal to energise their new and totally changed life direction.

It is made with the sun method only using the flowers.

Flowering Currant (*Ribes Sanguineum 'Pulborough Scarlet'*)

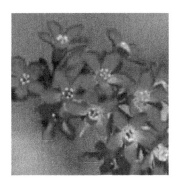

This essence is for those who have lost heart, but keep going. Often, they feel that they are facing inevitable defeat.

They feel despondent. The real problem with animals in this state is that they do not recognise their own strength and the power of their insight. Often, they are so frightened or intimidated that, like children, they try to hide their faces, hoping it will all go away. Flowering Currant will help your animal with the discovery of personal power, thereby bringing the confidence back into their life. It is only by fearlessly looking directly at opposing forces that we can see how to deflect or overcome them. Even when things are not so extreme, Flowering Currant can be very helpful. It encourages animals to let go of fears and to open up to the reality of their present situation.

It is made with the sun method using only the flowers.

Forsythia *(Oleacea Intermedia)*

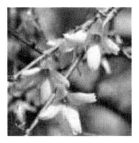

Forsythia helps us open up to our spiritual nature, bringing joy and a sense of freedom in that realisation.

Forsythia will allow your animal to open up to their true spiritual nature. Forsythia essence is complex; firstly, it will allow your animal to let go of old rooted behaviours. It is as if it squeezes your animal through a narrow tube, expelling anything that they no longer need. Secondly, it will allow your animal to see that there are many realities in the spiritual dimension. When something is misunderstood, it can generate fears and anxiety which Forsythia can reduce.

It is made with the sun method using only the flowers.

Foxglove *(Digitalis Purpurea)*

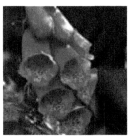

This essence is for those who feel confused in life and suffer from woolly thinking. Foxglove helps to bring the needed stillness to the mind.

Foxglove is the essence for animals that become despondent and lose their drive. They have lost their direction and get frustrated. Foxglove will help your animal to see things more clearly and will reduce the emotional entanglement of the problem which will result in a quieter mind and bring clarity to any situation.

It is made with the sun method using only the flowers.

Fuji Cherry *(Prunus Incisa)*

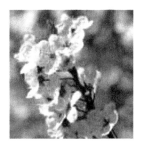

This essence helps us to relax and take life less seriously. It is the key essence for personal tranquillity.

Fuji Cherry is the key essence for developing a calm and quiet mind within your animal. It makes sense that a tense mind will create a tense body. The Fuji Cherry will help the mind to quieten, bringing in a sense of calmness and detachment to replace previous worries and difficulties that your animal may be experiencing. It will allow your animal to be detached from any dominating experiences that may surround them. An animal with a restless mind will often pace and be unable to settle. This essence would also make an excellent sleep tonic as it is literally calmness in a bottle.

It is made with the sun method using only the flowers.

Giant Bellflower *(Campanula Latifolia)*

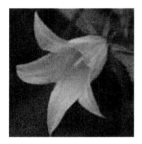

This essence is the clarion call for change. It is the catalyst for action where old habit patterns have been holding us back.

The Giant Bellflower is unique in the way it is created. Made with the sun method using only the flowers, the seed head is then floated separately in vodka for the same length of time. The two are mixed together to make the mother tincture. It is a catalyst for ringing out the old and ringing in the new. Like humans, animals often find it difficult to embrace change and often get stuck in old attitudes and patterns. The Giant Bellflower will help to smooth their path when change is necessary, and indeed inevitable. Whenever there is a major change in your animal's life, such as a new owner, home or illness, consider this flower. It is a flower that is not easily ignored as it rises above all other vegetation. In just the same way, the essence of the Bellflower is beautiful and not to be ignored when it sounds its clarion call.

Made with the sun method using only the flowers. The seed head is then floated separately in vodka in the sun for the same length of time. The two are mixed together to make the mother tincture.

Greater Celandine *(Chelidonium Majus)*

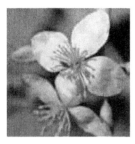

This essence encourages us to go deeper into our consciousness – to discover more of what we really are.

Greater Celandine is for animals who fear their spiritual nature. Many animals have put up, however unwittingly, a mental block between themselves and the source of their existence. This essence has the property of gradually dissolving the inner barriers that have been erected between the left and right hemispheres of the brain. As these dissolve, the intuitive mind can take its rightful place as part of a composite whole. Animals are far more connected to the spiritual realm than we are but with the excessive chemicals in their environment, from floor cleaners to chemical odour sprays, their spiritual connection to mother earth is in constant threat of being eroded.

It is made with the sun method using only the flowers.

Hairy Sedge *(Luzula Campestris)*

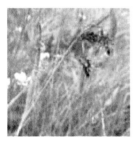

This essence is for those who worry and find it difficult to keep their minds in the present moment. This inattention can result in poor memory.

This essence is for those animals who find difficulty in living in the present and who tend to dwell either in the past or in possible futures. The Reiki precepts impact in the same way as this essence as they encourage you to live in the 'now'. Not to dwell on the past or to worry about the future. This essence would be excellent for animals with Alzheimer's disease as it will aid memory and any fears associated with the lack of memory. As our animals age, they are equally showing the same illnesses as their human friends. Dementia is now a common ailment among our four-legged pets.

It is made with the sun method only using the flowers.

Hairy Sedge was originally misidentified. Its correct Latin name is above and its correct common name is Field Woodrush.

Hawkweed *(Hieracium Vulgatum)*

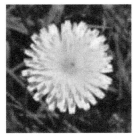

This essence is for those times when we have little confidence in ourselves because life seems to be so uncertain.

Hawkweed is for the type of despair caused by a lack of self-confidence. This is not the Blackthorn pit of despair, but more of a feeling of having lost touch with one's original roots. A feeling of being ungrounded. Animals who lose their confidence are often desperate to please their owners but with lack of confidence, it often leads to depressive emotional feelings. Hawkweed will allow your animal to be reborn into their confident former self and bring balance and harmony back into their life. This beautiful yellow flower resonates with your animal's solar plexus, bolstering self-assurance and happiness.

It is made with the sun method using only flowers.

Heath Bedstraw *(Galium Saxatile)*

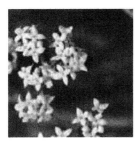

This essence is for helping us to find inner stillness and the peace of tranquil meditation states.

Heath Bedstraw supports your animal to let go of any tension caused by personal change in their life. When anything changes, it can cause your animal to be stressed and to naturally cling on to their old behaviours. Heath Bedstraw grows on the moors and the essence is made from the tiny white flower, which helps to underpin and support your animal as they undertake change. When animals embark on a new path in life they can feel very vulnerable when their circumstances change. Heath Bedstraw will help your animal to relax and will support your animal through any major time of change in their life. It is often a very helpful essence when given as a support to other essences that are actively promoting change.

It is made with the sun method using only the flowers.

Himalayan Blue Poppy (*Meconopsis Grandis*)

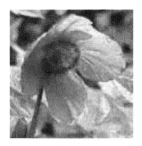

This is the essence of spiritual lineage. To fulfil our potential in this lifetime, we need to build on strengths gained in the past. It furthers insight and psychic skills.

The Himalayan Poppy will help your animal to return to their original blueprint. Each animal enters the world with different characteristics, many of which could be genetic or from previous lifetimes. These characteristics are their heritage, their original genetic make-up. If they are to fulfil their potential in this lifetime, then it will be important that they build on strengths gained from the past. This essence will give your animal insight so that they can make the right choices. This is the essence for the spiritual warrior, the person dedicated to being 'valiant for truth'. The more we can understand about this wonderful universe and about our own purpose in life, the more fulfilled we will become and the more we will be able to help others.

It is made with the sun method using only the flowers.

Holly Leaf (*Ilex Aquifolium*)

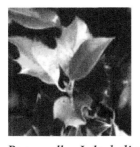

This essence helps us to see things as they really are and therefore to let go of pent-up anger and bitterness.

Holly Leaf is the key remedy for anger and resentment – it mirrors your animal's difficulties in its sharp defensive prickles. It is very difficult to say that animals get angry. Personally, I do believe that there are situations which cause them some annoyance. Animals that retaliate to being pushed and poked to the point of lashing out are showing a healthy tipping point of 'enough is enough'. After the cause of anger has dissipated they will go back to doing what they were doing before. However, if for any reason they are unable to deal with the anger as it arises, it will be held within the mind and body and emerge as bitterness, which in animals can manifest as resentment. Holly Leaf essence acts in several ways. First, it acts as a protection for the animal so they do not react instantaneously to provocation. It will give the animal a space of contemplation so they can assess the situation. Secondly, it takes the sting out of the situation by deflecting any intended desire to hurt them. Like the watery shine on the holly leaf which prevents things sticking to it, this essence enables the animal to be less sensitive to the provocation of others. In addition, the sharp spines of the Holly act as a protection, showing others that it is not wise to provoke them as they may well be hurt themselves. In animal terms, I like the fact that this essence can offer protection to your animal. It can protect your animal from harsh words and thoughts.

It is made with the alcohol method using the leaves before the berries come out.

Honesty *(Lunaria Annua)*

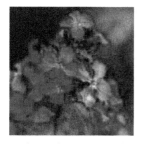

This essence is for bringing openness and receptivity where previously there were subversive negative characteristics.

Honesty, as the name suggests, is for a lack of openness and receptivity. It can help animals when there is an imbalance of Yin and Yang in the brain perhaps caused by a dominant owner.

When the Yang side of the brain is suppressed, the Yin side of the brain will then use this side of the brain in an attempt to assert themselves, as they feel resentful about how they were treated. When the female and masculine Yin and Yang are not in balance, your animal will be out of sorts. This flower essence would be good for animals who suffer with travel sickness and at any time there is imbalance, whether it be physical or emotional.

It is made with the sun method using only the flowers.

Honeysuckle *(Lonicera Periclymemum)*

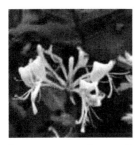

This essence helps us to become more open to the world around us.

The wild yellow Honeysuckle growing in our hedgerows possesses very strong healing properties. It has an exquisite scent which is strongest in the late evening. This essence will encourage your animal to make their fragrance known to others. Sadness and loneliness isolate your animal from other animals and people. So, your animal turns inwards and becomes increasingly closed to the positive aspects of the world around them. The walls that are built during periods of sadness and loneliness are natural, but unfortunately are often very counter-productive as they close off your animal to the world around them. Honeysuckle helps to ease the pain in their heart, enabling them to open up. Through this opening up, loving help will often flow in their direction because they will then become less defensive. Honeysuckle has two properties. First, it brings ease and comfort to their heart, Second, it helps us to pull down the built-up walls that your animal has erected between you and other animals.

It is made with the sun method using only the flowers.

Indian Balsam *(Impatiens Glandulifera)*

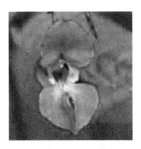

This essence brings quietness and peace to an overactive and disturbed mind.

Indian Balsam brings quietness and healing to minds that are disturbed, helping your animal to distance themselves from thoughts that are causing them distress. There can be little more distressing than a mind caught up in endless mind-loops that just will not stop. You will often see your animal pacing and feeling very unsettled. Under such circumstances there can be no peace because as soon as the mind starts to quieten, new looping thoughts arise. Indian Balsam prevents such thoughts from reinforcing themselves by reducing the emotional tensions in the mind. This essence would be excellent for stereotypical behaviour such as the weaving behaviour of a horse. It helps the mind to steady down to a point where they can once more take charge of their thinking. I strongly believe that when animals are distressed they literally start to live on their nerves and every new situation becomes very stressful to them.

It is made with the sun method using only the flowers.

Ivy *(Hedera Helix)*

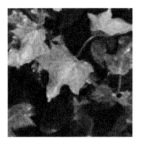

This essence helps us to be strongly rooted in the world when we feel uprooted by the forces around us.

Ivy is the essence to ground your animal when situations of shock arise that may make your animal space out and even lose the will to live. It may be that the shock of a bad accident has made your animal lose touch with reality, to a point where they give up. In such circumstances your animal will need an essence that will help them to root back in the physical world, to feel secure and loved. This is where Ivy can help. Ivy mirrors the properties that your animal is looking for. Ivy is a survivor and holds the key to endurance.

It is made with the alcohol method using only the young leaves.

Larch *(Larix Decidua)*

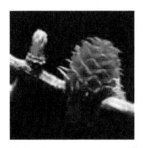

This essence encourages the intuitive side of our nature to expand and take its rightful place in our life.

Larch is the essence for awakening the true power of Yin within your animal. Yin represents many things. It is the shadow side of a mountain, the depths rather than the heights.
It is the receptive side of their nature – the intuitive. It is about love, compassion and nurturing. It is soft but powerful in its softness. In many ways it is femininity in its purest form – yet it is far more than that. Yin accepts rather than confronts. Yin wisdom because Yang fears the wisdom of Yin, it tends to dominate Yin. It covers this up by pretending that intuition (which means inner tuition) is just wishful

thinking. The essence of Larch (made from the red male catkins in the spring) is a powerful activator of Yin qualities. This essence would be excellent when there is a lot of male testosterone in the air, such as in dogs that are not neutered. When there is too much masculine energy, battles will be fought; this essence will lower the tension within the house hold so that balance of energies can be created.

It is made with the alcohol method using the red catkins of early spring.

Leopardsbane *(Dornicum Pardalianches)*

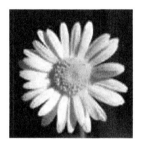

This essence is for those who are at a major change point in their lives. They may feel as if they are living on a knife-edge.

Leopardsbane is the essence for animals that are living on a knife-edge and seeing this in your animal can be very distressing. The negative aspect of the Leopardsbane characteristic is that it can lead to serious depression and even to suicidal thoughts. Because of the powerful emotions generated in such states, there is often a real problem with addiction to the feelings of negativity. Animals in this state are often shut down as they are trapped in their own suffering. Leopardsbane is useful in two ways: first, in lessening the attachment to emotional extremes; second, in allowing the perceptions to broaden.

It is made with the sun method using only the flowers.

Lesser Stitchwort *(Stellaria Graminea)*

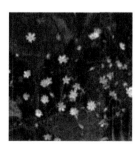

This essence is for 'possession', i.e. for those whose behaviour is dominated by others or by strongly held ideas.

Lesser Stitchwort is the essence for animals who need to escape from the thought patterns and influences that possess them. The things that possess them can be many and various: they may be attitudes and opinions that they have come to believe in;

someone may be trying to dominate them; it may even be an obsession with objects. Sometimes animals can be obsessed with a toy, which if lost or parted with makes them extremely anxious. Lesser Stitchwort works in two ways. First, it helps to dissolve their attachment with objects, events and people. These greatly restrict their freedom of action. Second, it acts, like a guiding star, to illuminate the path ahead. The pretty white delicate flowers offer encouragement when it is difficult for your animal to see the light at the end of the tunnel.

It is made with the sun method using only the flowers.

Lichen *(Marchantia Polymorpha L)*

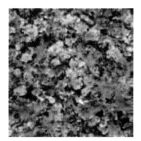

This essence is to help us feel at ease and at one with our surroundings.

Lichens are strange plants composed of two different species living together in an interlocked relationship. The essence of Lichen mirrors this, but in a rather different manner. When you look at life at a deeper level you realise that everything is made up of energy and that everything is connected. Another name for this is the 'universe'. Animals are far more spiritually advanced than humans and they realise that they are part of the universe and the universe is a part of them. When that relationship becomes strained and the universe becomes misaligned, there is disconnection. This essence is about bonding, and will help animals who find it difficult to bond with humans and any other species.

It is made with sun method using a piece of the whole plant.

Lilac *(Syringa Vulgaris 'Massena')*

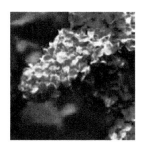

This essence is for those whose personal development has been stunted by dominant influences, usually in childhood adolescence.

The Lilac flower is for those animals who have failed to develop fully and blossom in their life and whose personal growth has therefore been stunted. This may have been caused by a dominant owner. The result of such domination is very oppressing to the animal. Lilac encourages an opening up and leads to a more confident animal. Your animal realises that all is not lost and that they have simply been hibernating. Unblocking locked-in energies can give remarkably rapid personal growth, rather like plant growth in the spring. Often Lilac animals have difficulty in accepting their own worth and potential. Opening the door of the cage and looking out into a much wider world can feel threatening. Love and support are needed to help support your animal through such a major change. We are talking here about true love, not sentimentality.

It is made with the sun method using only the flowers.

Lily of the Valley *(Convallaria Majalis)*

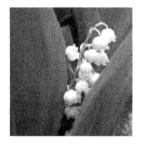

This essence is for yearning; for those who have been blocked by desiring the unattainable.

The Lily of the Valley holds the answers for items that are seemingly unobtainable in your animal's life. It is like searching for the Holy Grail and never finding it, however hard. This yearning causes a sense of desperation until the object of desire is achieved. It is like a heart burn that will not go away. The answer lies in giving up the search! Some animals have a fixation and are literally fixed onto an object or target and lose a sense of everything around them. Lily of the Valley will allow a more relaxed approach to guarding of any kind.

It is made with the sun method using only the flowers.

Magnolia *(Magnolia x Loebneri 'Leonard Messel')*

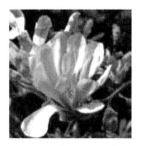

This essence is for unconditional love. This essence helps to bring and awaken within us the energies of love and compassion.

The Magnolia flower is associated with the double-edged sword of love and compassion.

Unconditional love is not necessarily pleasant; it has nothing of the sentimental aspects that so often pass for love. Indeed, it can be very disturbing to be on the receiving end of its attentions! It will not let us go. Love is the most powerful emotion and can heal many things but when the love is unhealthy it can be all consuming. Animals are of pure heart and live in the Magnolia state; when their life is empty of love and compassion this essence will show them that love does, indeed, conquer all. Magnolia helps your animal to go forward into those expanded realms with courage and fortitude.

It is made with the sun method using only the flowers.

Mahonia *(Mahonia Aquifolium)*

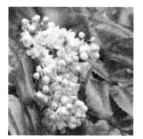

This essence helps us to let go of our illusions and thus see into the true nature of things.

Mahonia helps to free your animal from the fear of their negative potential. When the burden of fear lifts, there is a great release of the energy which has been trapped by the negative thoughts. That energy will then activate unconditional love within the Heart Chakra, love that has been blocked by the fears of the past. This is a very uplifting essence that can be a great help to all animals who feel that they are inadequate.

It is made with the sun method using only the flowers.

Marigold *(Calendula Officianalis)*

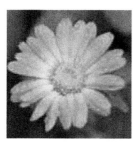

This essence is for where there is a rigid materialistic approach to life, often with a total denial of the psychic and spiritual dimensions.

Marigold is the essence for the animal who has largely blocked their feminine sensitivity. Every animal needs balance, as too much masculine energy feeds a fearful ego. Whereas the Aqueous Bracken personality is merely suppressing their sensitivity, the Marigold personality has gone one stage further. Marigold is therefore particularly useful for all those animals who have largely blocked the light from their feminine side. It helps to dissipate the fear of the feminine aspects and gently encourages the growth of positive insight.

It is made with the sun method using only the flowers.

Marsh Thistle *(Cirsium Palustre)*

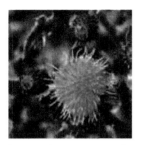

This remedy is for those locked in the past; for those who cling on to old, outmoded patterns of thought and behaviour.

Marsh Thistle is for those animals who have become locked in the past. Animals like routine, they like to know when they are going to be fed, walked or ridden. Routine has its advantages but it also causes a fear or suspicion if the exercise is not carried out.

Marsh Thistle helps the fear of newness to fade but allows the change to take place gently. In this case, everything new is welcomed, however inappropriate it may be. This essence would be perfect in situations of change, for example when training an animal who may otherwise find it difficult to learn new things and be overwhelmed in the process

Marsh Thistle is the remedy for all those animals who are trapped in routine attitudes and situations. It is about being open to newness and change and welcoming those changes as they occur.

It is made with the sun method using only the flowers.

Meadow Rue *(Thalictrum Dipterocarpum)*

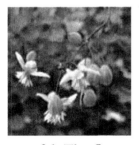

This essence is for discerning what is worth striving for in our life and what is unhealthy. It brings clarity to see where we need to be heading to fulfil our true purpose in life.

The Chinese Lesser Meadow Rue is the essence for discernment, showing your animal what will be. It is a tall plant and very fine and graceful. The flowers are small but incredibly beautiful, the petals a violet-purple with striking creamy-white anthers and stamens. The graceful energy of this flower teaches your animal about judgement and self-seeking for what is in their best interests. It is the flower of calmness and balance and it will allow your animal to live their life with grace and poise in a difficult world. It is the flower for service but at the same time it will not allow your animal to be a doormat.

It is made with the sun method using only the flowers.

Mediterranean Sage *(Salvia Fruticosa)*

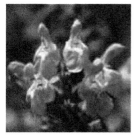

This essence is for the 'Earth' qualities of warmth, comfort and wisdom. Helps to catalyse insight from a firm earthed base.

The Mediterranean Sage represents all that is powerful within the element of Earth. It mirrors the energy and wisdom of the Mother Earth. It helps your animal to stay grounded and keeps them aware of all that is going on around them.

Mediterranean Sage has deep roots that grow deeply down into Mother Earth. This essence will bring qualities of steadfastness and dependability to your animal. It manages to grow where there seems to be little to nourish it. Sage has always been linked with wisdom, but the flower essence made from plants growing in wild mountainous areas has additional qualities. This essence brings warmth and comfort as well as quiet wisdom.

Sage essence also reflects the quality of stillness. The Earth element is very still, acting as a firm base for the other elements. Sage can help your animal to mirror this stillness within their own being, so that they can safely venture into other realms of reality. Animals need stability and they need to feel that they are connected to the earth.

It is made with the sun method using only the flowers.

Milk Thistle *(Sonchus Arvensis)*

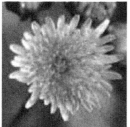

This remedy is for those who do not love themselves. Often they try to make up for this by trying to please others. The Milk Thistle essence relates to the chest area of your animal – in Eastern terms the heart centre, the heart ki, all that is love. (Heart Chakra.)

For many animals this is a vulnerable place because it is where they experience fear as well as love. Animals are continually being pushed to their limits and often find themselves being put into a Rescue Centre because their owner is unable to cope with their behaviour. Animals must learn how to love and trust again and this can be a very difficult thing for them to do after they have experienced such abuse. Fear can suppress love, yet love can overcome fear. This essence will allow the animal to love and to be loved.

Milk Thistle encourages animals to open up to love and let go of the fears that are restricting them. They will then begin to understand that the world itself is a loving environment.

It is made with the sun method using only the flowers.

Monk's Hood *(Aconitum Napellus)*

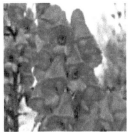

This essence is for difficulties of long standing that have their roots in the distant past. It helps to bring one up-to-date.

The Monk's Hood flower essence is for long-standing difficulties, the roots of which lie in the past.

Such chronic difficulties show that problems have been carried forward rather than being resolved at the time when they originally occurred. Any trauma that has happened in the 'socialisation' period for an animal is often very difficult to let go of. This essence will help to heal past traumas and it will help them to understand that it is okay now to let them go. Monk's Hood gently helps them to see things of the past as they really were, and not the fearful memories that they think they were.

It is made with the sun method using only the flowers.

Moss *(Thytidiadelphus Squarrosus)*

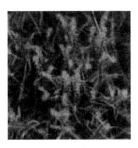

This essence is for those who fear freedom and lightness in their lives. Often it is a fear of dark spaces within the being.

Moss is the essence for those animals who fear the dark spaces within themselves. Interestingly enough, my cat Reuben chose this essence when he was scared of a black cat that was coming into our garden. Some of these fears may be from the past, so come with more of a more dogged intensity. There is something very untoward, murky and very dark that instils these deep anxieties. Moss helps to show that fears about the subconscious are only paper tigers – shadows that disappear when light is shed on them. It is fear that prevents the light of insight from entering the mind, and fear is therefore responsible for the dark spaces.

It is made with the alcohol method using the whole plant.

Nasturtium *(Tropaeolum Majus)*

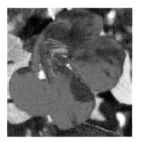

This essence is for those who know that they need to make changes in their life, but seem to be unable to make the first move.

The Nasturtium essence is for those animals who find it difficult to cope with change. Although they may wish to do so, they feel unable to start the change process. There are two factors needed for this to happen, and Nasturtium helps with both. The first is having sufficient energy to initiate the change. The second is a recognition of the need to let go of the attitudes and fears that will otherwise inhibit the change process. In fact, it is usually this latter factor that is the key problem. Change can be difficult for animals that become set in their routine, such as walks and the brand of food that they eat. Nasturtium encourages change, growth and a bright new future. It will help your animal to see it as a positive experience and not one to dread.

It is made with the sun method using only the flowers.

Norway Maple *(Acer Platinoides)*

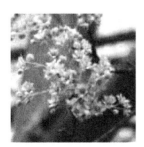

This essence helps us understand more about our true nature, freeing up our mind so that we can more easily enter other levels of consciousness.

The Norway Maple will help your animal to see the world more clearly, by offering them insight in to problems that they may not have considered before. Norway Maple works to free up their consciousness so that that they no longer put blocks on what they are prepared to accept. It will entice your animal to develop an enquiring mind. It encourages them to go further and deeper to find solutions to problems that they may have not witnessed before. This essence would be excellent to use when there is training required of any animal, as it will allow them to see the whole picture and not just a specific part of it.

It is made with the sun method using only the yellowish-green flowers.

Oak *(Quercus Robur)*

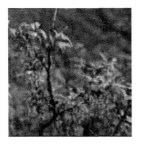

This essence imparts quiet inner strength and wisdom. It helps us to relax and to find our own strengths.

The mighty oak tree will help your animal if there is confusion, an overactive mind, or a lack of inner strength. It will help your animal to be rooted to the earth. The flowers of this tree are used to make the essence. Animals with an overactive mind will often be seen to be pacing and will be unable to settle. This essence would be useful in helping animals with stereotypical behaviour, as it will allow them to be strong and resilient.

It is made with the alcohol method using the female catkins.

Oriental Poppy *(Papaver Somniferum)*

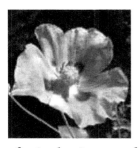

This essence alleviates the pain of addiction and helps to break up dependencies, whether they are in the mind, body or spirit.

Animals can also suffer with dependent behaviour, and as a result of that, have less freedom (they can't just leave). Some animals will 'sleep-walk' through their life, feeling a deep level of pain that is covered over by an addiction to an unhealthy habit. This habit could be the habit of clinging to a person, it could be attacking another animal or it could be eating something that makes them sick. It could be unseen – but an animal will display the 'same' behaviour, as though on auto-pilot, and that they are not in the present moment. They display the signs of a 'being' who is sleep-walking through life. And they do this to cover the extreme pain that they feel inside through an inherent need.

That is addiction. A behaviour that not just covers pain, but pushes it down.

The result of taking Oriental Poppy is to allow your animal to move beyond an addiction that covers pain. To alleviate that pain so that they can move on. When Oriental Poppy is needed, it is clear that more support with other essences would be necessary.

It is made with the sun method using only the flowers.

Oxalis *(Oxalis Pes-Caprae)*

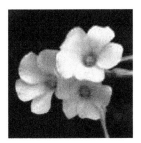

This essence is for things that 'have you by the throat' and seem so overpowering that there appears to be no way out.

This beautiful pure yellow flower is widespread in many parts of the world. It can be found in places as far apart as Bermuda and South Africa.

Communication among animals is very important as it contributes to survival of a species. It is especially important that animals find a way to express themselves with us, since they must often feel trapped by the difficulty involved in getting us to understand! Therefore animal communication is so precious and well worth investing in learning that skill. If they are deprived of this basic skill, then a whole array of other problems can creep in. Oxalis helps to unblock the energy in the Throat Chakra. As the throat area frees up, so then is the animal allowed to speak freely. Oxalis is especially important when your animal needs to find a way to express themselves to us. Since we cannot speak dog, cat or horse language, it makes sense that they must often feel trapped by the difficulty involved in getting us to understand!

It is made with the sun method using only the flowers.

Pine Cones *(Pinus Sylvestris)*

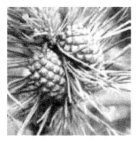

This essence is for those who are trapped by the authoritarian power of others, and feel unable to escape from them.

The essence of Pine Cones is for those animals who feel trapped by the authoritarian power of their owners and are unable to escape. They are trapped in a situation where they are continually being put down and shouted at, which leads to a source of inadequacy. There may be such a lack of self-confidence and a feeling of no worth. The world becomes a very frightening place leading them to live in a fearful energy. The Pine Cones essence helps your animal to break free from the thoughts of pleasing their owner and to be free from the chains of authority that hold them back.

It is made with the alcohol method using the very small cones (fruit of the tree) in spring. In this case, the cones are steeped for several weeks in alcohol.

Pink Purslane *(Montia Siberica)*

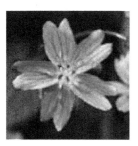

This essence is for those needing to expand their horizons and leave behind the limitations of the past.

Pink Purslane is the essence that relates to views of reality, the here and now and will allow your animal not to be easily influenced by those around them, whether that be their owner or other animals. When your animal follows the influences of others they are not truly following their own destiny. If your animal is uncertain and looks to you for guidance, this essence will give them insight into what the true answer may be. This beautiful small pink flower radiates the energy of compassion and understanding and is the flower of freedom.

It is made with the sun method using only the flowers.

Ragwort *(Senecio Jacobaea)*

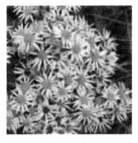

This essence is to break the power of obsessive thoughts that keep on endlessly looping round and round.

Ragwort will help your animal to tackle problems at their roots. It interrupts the endless looping thoughts that would otherwise keep your animal in a constant loop of anxiety. Animals in this modern world are often exhibiting signs of obsessive behaviour; this can include excessive grooming, weaving and crib biting. Ragwort has two properties that can help your animal. Firstly, it works to remove the emotional kick that they get from obsessive thoughts. The stereotypical behaviour helps to relieve stress and serves no other purpose. Secondly it is a strong, tough plant. That quality of strength can support your animal during a period of change while they adjust to having a much quieter mind. It may seem surprising, but a quiet mind can feel somewhat distressing if your animal has become accustomed to the constant mind chatter of obsessive thoughts.

It is made with the sun method using only the flowers.

Red Clover *(Trifolium Pratense)*

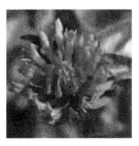

This essence is for those who are blocked off by fear of their own emotional nature.

Red Clover is for animals who are emotionally blocked off and they are suppressing their emotions. Red Clover gently encourages the emotional side to emerge. It is important that this change is gradual so that the changes can be integrated without stress.

Here the problem is usually due to a largely blocked-off right (intuitive) brain function. Red Clover encourages communication between the two sides of the personality. The left (logical) brain will then begin to allow and trust the activities of the right brain and finally rejoice that it has such an amazing partner to work with!

It is made with the sun method using only the flowers.

Red Frangipani *(Frangipani Plumeria Rubra)*

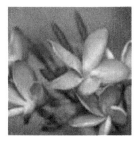

The essence is for awakening. It reunites us with the true source of our being, which lies beyond the spiritual dimension. It brings joy and new levels of perception and confidence.

This beautiful fragrant flower has the power to reunite your animal with the source of their very being. Their true essence can also be described as their soul. The ego knows that in such experience, it will inevitably begin to dissolve and disappear. This creates deep fears. It has been likened to the fear that a raindrop could feel when it falls towards a river, where it knows it will merge and disappear into a greater unity. The soul is the nonphysical existence of your animal and lights up their true purpose and destiny. This essence is about lightness of living and clarity of vision. It brings joy and ease, true self-confidence and new levels of perception.

It is made with the sun method using only the flowers.

Red Poppy *(Papaver Rhoeas)*

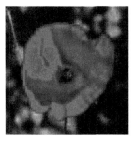

This essence is to help us leave our limitations behind and to find our true energy and power.

The Red Poppy helps to stabilise the 'fire' energy of your animal. An animal with too much fire energy will be very excitable and over-exuberant. The element of fire is both creative and destructive. It is the force behind all that they do: too little fire and they become ineffective, too much and they become destructive.

Red Poppy helps to stabilise their fire energy, preventing them from becoming excessively angry or turning their anger inwards. It will help them to let go of the anger so that they can assess difficult situations more accurately. When animals are filled with rage, they cannot see clearly and are more likely to lash out and possibly hurt another animal or themselves. Red Poppy is thus a very positive healing essence that can bring much balance to any animal that is out of sorts.

It is made with the sun method using only the flowers.

Rhododendron *(Rhododendron Ponticum)*

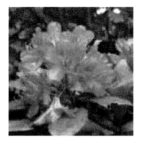

This essence is for those who lack flexibility and keep trying to push through blind alleys.

Rhododendron is for those animals who have not learned how to solve problems. They may become overloaded so that a solution is too difficult to understand. They find it hard to stand back and look carefully at the whole situation. With such a detached viewpoint, your animal may use the wrong methods to achieve the end result. Rhododendron will help your animal to see the wider context and to ask questions about the situation. Maybe the problem is insolvable and they keep making the same mistakes. Rhododendron will help them to see the answer more clearly and not to waste time on things that have no purpose.

It is made with the sun method using only the flowers.

Rosebay Willowherb *(Chamaenerion Angustifolium)*

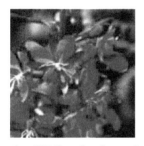

This essence is for times of major upheaval when we feel disoriented and lost.

Rosebay Willowherb is the essence for your animal when they are affected by the winds of change. There is a complete lack of earth energy, so they can be easily influenced by the world around them. Like the down of the Willowherb in the autumn, they are blown hither and thither by the forces that surround them. They feel very unsure of themselves and of the world around. The essence of Willowherb helps them to root themselves firmly to the earth and their present situation. It gives them stability and strength. Only when they are stable and quiet can they truly evaluate the situation that they find themselves in.

It is made with the sun method using only the flower.

Round-Headed Leek *(Allium Sphaerocephalon L)*

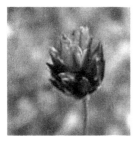

This essence is for unknown difficulties stemming from childhood, particularly when other essences have been ineffective.

The Round Headed Leek is a tiny member of the onion family and it grows in Cyprus. The essence made from it is very useful for those animals who have difficulties relating to problems from when they were young. The problem is buried within their subconscious and often they are not able to work out exactly what the problem is. With this unknowingness, it does not allow them to deal with the problem. Hence it can have a negative effect on their future self. Here the Round-Headed essence helps to neutralise the forces (usually of fear) that are holding old patterns within the unconscious areas of the mind. Once they can see these patterns and clearly identify them, then it is much easier to release them. The Round Headed Leek helps to bring those old repressed energies to the surface.

It is made with the sun method using only the flowers.

Sacred Lotus *(Nelumbo Nucifera)*

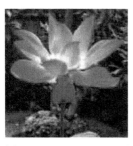

This is a powerful essence to open the heart to the love of the Universe and the Divine.

The sacred lotus is a very beautiful flower which encourages the blossoming of personal growth. It helps to open the heart to the love of the Universe and the Divine. It is a very spiritual flower and will allow your animal to blossom. Are animals spiritual? I personally believe that they are far more spiritually aware than we are. They are connected to the earth and understand the cycles of the seasons and the moon. All flowers take time to grow and blossoming comes from living on the physical earth. Like all flower essences, the intelligence within the essence knows what your animal needs at any time. We cannot force progress. This essence encourages the blossoming of your animal's personal growth. This beautiful essence was made using the fully developed seed pod and a photograph of the lotus in flower. The water was energised in the sun with the photograph. Underneath the bowl, the pod was floated in vodka in the glass bowl and left in the sun. The two were then combined.

Scabious *(Knautia Arvensis)*

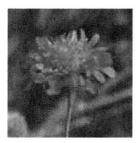

This essence is for healing us when we need gentleness and quiet support.

Scabious initiates the healing process after serious shock or trauma. Shock is a complex process and it can arise from a variety of causes, and presents in a multitude of ways. This essence will bring comfort to the shocked mind, as an animal in this state will find it difficult to cope and often their whole body will shut down. A shocked mind can easily inhibit the healing that would otherwise naturally take place. Scabious gently helps your animal to accept what has happened, whatever the apparent consequences, so that their distress does not block the natural healing.

It is made with the sun method using only the flowers.

Scarlet Pimpernel *(Anagallis Arvensis)*

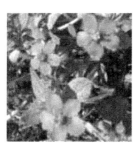

This essence is for those who are emotionally trapped by others, often with a psychic dependence.

Scarlet Pimpernel is a useful essence for animals who are emotionally entangled with another person or animal. This happens quite often between the animal and owner. There are two states the flower deals with – either being obsessed or being 'possessed' by someone else. In either case they are unable to break free, even though they may realise that the relationship is unsatisfactory and probably very bad for them. Scarlet Pimpernel works at a hidden level, enabling your animal to disconnect the ties that bind them, and to gain sufficient power to break free.

It is made with the sun method using only the flowers.

Sea Campion *(Silene Maritima)*

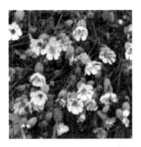

This essence is for separation in early childhood and its consequent insecurity and fears. It stimulates loving, protective energies.

Sea Campion is the essence for those animals who have suffered separation early on in their lives. Whilst this is most frequently due to a separation from the mother, a separation from the protective male energy of the father can also cause trauma. All animals need to have a close bond with their mothers. This is the most important time in an animal's life, as this is when they are learning the skills of how to be the animal they were meant to be. Animals in the wild would instinctively be with their mother for a much longer period than they are in the modern world. This would offer a close bond with their mothers during the early stages of life. This builds up a sense of security and of being cared for and loved. That in turn gives a strong base for the infant to grow up from, feeling secure in the world in which it finds itself. Animals have a really hard time if they are taken away from their mothers and siblings far too early. This leads to animals who have no sense of who they are or how they are able to communicate with their own species. They often live in a constant state of fear, as the world they live in is a very scary place. They have not had enough time to learn how to be a dog, cat or horse, which leads to deep-rooted feelings of fear. Sea Campion therefore is a flower that helps your animal to be rooted to the earth so they can find their true roots, which will allow them to feel peace and contentment.

It grows on bleak windswept cliffs that are battered by the winter storms, yet still blossoms in the spring. Sea Campion is a 'return to the earth' flower, helping to bring ease to the insecure heart.

It is made with the sun method using only the flowers.

Sheep's Sorrel *(Rumex Acetosella)*

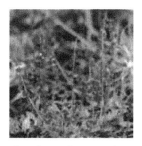

This essence is for the bitterness that arises when we feel that life is being desperately unfair to us.

Sheep's Sorrel is for bitterness, the type of bitterness that arises when we feel that life is unfair. It is for the anguished cry of, "Why should this have happened to me?" Animals that have been mistreated can feel resentful and bitter towards people or other animals such as caused by a bereavement or separation. Sheep's Sorrel will help your animal to accept what has happened. It encourages your animal to let go of bitterness and to move forward into a new and changed future.

It is made using the alcohol method.

Siberian Spruce *(Picea Omorika)*

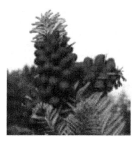

This remedy is for those whose 'male' energy is lacking, producing frustration and a lack of clarity.

The Siberian Spruce is for those animals whose 'male' energy is low. Being assertive means you can express yourself. Being assertive is a way that your animal can communicate to other animals or people. It does not mean 'aggressive', it is about being responsible for their behaviour.

Sensitive animals, whose 'feminine' aspect is dominant, often have difficulties in dealing with the Yang side of their nature. It is the opposite of the Red Clover personality. They are equally unbalanced but in opposite directions. This essence offers a firm unshakeable grounding energy, and Siberian Spruce points the way to this.

It is made using the alcohol method.

Single Snowdrop *(Galanthus Nivalis)*

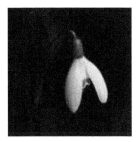

This essence is for breaking through to new levels of consciousness. It helps to bring insight and support during such times.

The Single Snowdrop flowers in late winter when the snow and ice carpets the ground. Its beautiful flower head pokes its way up through the ground and signals the start of new life. It is for those animals who are experiencing difficulties in breaking through old, habitual patterns of behaviour. They may feel under threat so they react negatively to remove that threat. The net result is that efforts to change positively are continually being subverted. Single Snowdrop helps to reveal the joyful potential of a true and wider vision. Old negative set ways can then be seen for what they really are.

It is made using the alcohol method.

Soapwort *(Saponaria Ocymoides)*

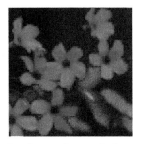

This essence is for use where there is bewilderment and lack of vision. It is for the 'what the hell am I doing here?' type of feeling.

Soapwort is the essence that is needed when your animal is bewildered, confused and they feel that they are trapped. The confusion could be caused by a trauma of any kind and can lead to physical distress. The loss of the old patterns can be a time of upset and stress, when the new has not yet fully emerged. It is in this personal 'void' that many deep positive changes can take place. Soapwort prevents your animal from falling back into these old ways. It can be viewed as helping to wash away the past negative influences and providing love and encouragement for embracing the new.

It is made using the alcohol method.

Solomon's Seal *(Polygonatum Multiflorum)*

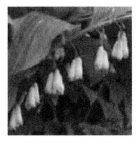

This essence is for the busy mind. This remedy helps bring quietness and detachment.

Solomon's Seal is the essence for those animals that feel overwhelmed. This could be a situation, an illness, or something more. They may be overwhelmed by a demanding owner or stressful training programme. This essence will bring a sense of calmness back into your animal's life. With a quietened mind your animal will be able to rest, allowing their body to heal.

It is made using the alcohol method.

Speedwell *(Veronica Chamaedrys)*

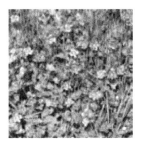

This essence increases powers of insight whilst preventing us from becoming emotionally entangled with what we perceive.

Speedwell will offer your animal insight in a very natural way. Speedwell gives your animal clarity of vision. This essence will also help your animal to be grounded and not to be persuaded to change the direction that they are going in. Having a good sense of clarity and vision comes into play when animals are unable to make clear choices and sway like the trees in the wind as to which will be the best way forward. Speedwell will show the problems in a way that they can be easily solved and resolved.

It is made using the alcohol method.

Spotted Orchid *(Dactylorhiza Fuchsii)*

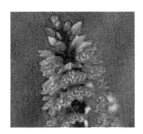

This essence is to help us overcome difficulties and blocks on our path of personal growth.

The Spotted Orchid will help your animal when the question is asked: 'Where do I go from here?' Animals have a great sense of direction, as it is a key survival mechanism. They like to be able to calculate the way forward and the best escape route. Spotted Orchid can provide support and guidance, sometimes pointing the way out through a complex maze that they need to explore. It will shine a light but they must do all of the hard work to get there.

It is made using the alcohol method.

Spring Squill *(Scilla Verna)*

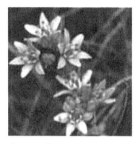

This essence is to achieve freedom after a breakthrough. It helps us to soar like a bird, finding our own true path in limitless space.

Spring Squill offers a space of freedom to your animal. It offers them a space of self-confidence and joy. Learning new concepts can often be very daunting for animals, as they may feel pressure from the owner to succeed. This essence will offer them the answers. Without that insight, their fears and attitudes may well paint it as a dark and fearsome place, to endure or to escape from. Spring Squill will help your animal to see more widely and deeply into the true nature of reality.

It is made using the alcohol method.

Star of Bethlehem *(Ornithogalum Arabicum)*

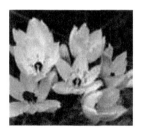

This is the key essence for reducing the effects of shock and trauma to the whole system.

Star of Bethlehem is used as the basic shock essence, taking the initial negative reaction out of the system. Animals that go into shock will have a physical shutdown of their whole system. Shock can be caused by a multitude of incidents, from a car accident to the loss of an owner or friend. When an animal is shocked the whole of their body's nerve system is severely upset. The initial shock reaction affects all the cells in the body and completely disrupts the body's energies. Indeed, animals often die more from shock than they do from injury in severe accidents.

On a deeper level, shock will affect your animal's will to live. This essence will help the animal's mind to immediately let go of the traumatic experience, allowing the body to heal and recover from the trauma. Always use whenever there is sudden shock in your animal's life.

It is made using the alcohol method.

Sumach *(Rhus Typina)*

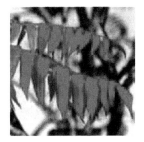

This essence is for those who ignore their own potential for fear of loss of their old identities.

Sumach is the essence for animals who lack confidence so never reach their full potential. They do not like to go outside their comfort zone as this is where they feel safest. They love to follow the same routine as this takes the least work. When you live in a world of mediocrity, reaching the height's full potential seems like a very difficult place to get to. This essence will show your animal that there is no hiding place and that it takes far less energy to accept what one is than waste energy in trying to oppose it.

It is made using the alcohol method.

Thrift *(Armeria Maritima)*

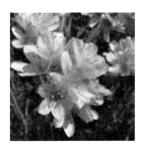

This essence is for helping to open up to psychic sensitivity, but keeping the person firmly grounded at the same time.

Thrift essence is the essence for being grounded and offers protection to your animal from other influences. Animals are energy sponges and will pick up and mirror the emotional problems of their owners. Carrying the emotional baggage of their owner becomes a great weight until they too take on their owner's symptoms and fears. Like a tree without roots, it will topple over and crash to the earth once it meets maturity. This essence will give your animal stability so they can be strongly 'earthed' and protected from their owner's energy.

It is made with the sun method using only the flowers.

Trailing St John's Wort *(Hypericum Humifusum)*

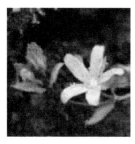

This essence is for helping us when our life has been irrevocably changed.

The Trailing St John's Wort is a pretty yellow flower that is used for healing, especially when there is emotional tension and despair caused by grief. A sudden shock in your animal's life, such as a death of an animal or owner, can be very distressing to your animal. This essence will offer a vibrational hug which will soothe the changes forced upon your animal. Trailing St John's Wort works gently but powerfully to ease the situation that is causing your animal so much stress. It helps them to rebalance and to see that there is a way forward, a way that is far brighter than they might believe while they are immersed in the depths of their despair.

It is made using the alcohol method.

Tree Mallow *(Lavatera Thuringiaca)*

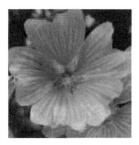

This essence is for those who have become addicted to being permanently busy.

Tree Mallow has healing and inspiring properties that will allow your animal to relax. An animal that is relaxed and centred will be well able to deal with any situation that comes their way. Tree Mallow will allow your animal to be present in this exact moment in time, with what exists in the 'now', and not be stressed by past fears that have prevented vital relaxation.

Tree Mallow will help your animal to centre their attention more easily in the present moment. In reality, that is the only real time that they ever really have.

It is made using the alcohol method.

Tufted Vetch (Vicia Cracca)

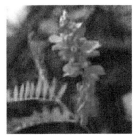

This essence is for sexual difficulties caused by an incorrect sexual self-image – usually due to childhood conditioning.

Tufted Vetch is the essence for sexual imbalance, when there is either too much masculine or too much feminine energy. It is then that there is no stability. If there is too much masculine energy this will lead to aggression and dominance of other animals or people, to a point that they may not consider all of the dangers ahead of them so therefore become reckless. If there is too much feminine energy, it will lead to manipulation and unfairness. Balance is always key as your animal will have strength and be of calm character.

It is made using the alcohol method.

Valerian (Valeriana Officinalis)

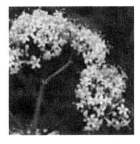

This essence is for those who have not had their need for love fulfilled in their childhood.

Valerian is the essence for the animal who feels like a lost soul and needs help and support. Instinctively as an owner one's heart goes out to animals like this – they seem so alone and helpless. Direct help is probably not needed at all. Usually the original cause is a problem from the past. They may feel unable to trust. Valerian encourages the development of self-love and self-esteem, and gradually reduces the need for external support.

It is made using the alcohol method.

Welsh Poppy (Meconopsis Cambrica)

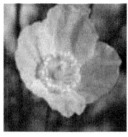

This essence is for those who have lost their fire and inspiration and become day-dreamers.

Welsh Poppy is for those animals who have lost their 'mojo'. It is those animals that have previously been energised and active, but whose life force energies have become dissipated and lethargic. Their survival instinct becomes less important and they find it difficult to be inspired, instead accepting whatever is laid in front of them even if the situation happens to be bad. Welsh Poppy helps to bring energy and inspiration back into their lives.

It is made using the alcohol method.

White Cherry (Prunus Taihaku)

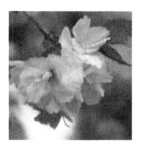

This essence helps past negative influences to lose their grip and be dissipated.

White Cherry is the essence for dissolving old cellular memories that are deep rooted. It will allow your animal to free themselves from old patterns and negative influences from the past.

Treating the emotion does not, however, solve the problem; unless the cause is removed, the emotional reaction will recur. These deeply rooted patterns from the past are imprinted in all of their cells, hence the instantaneous shock that can accompany some of these old energies when they are triggered. When an animal is held back by old behaviours and fears, they are unable to enjoy their present situation. Once these past fears are healed at a cellular level, your animal is no longer bound to them and can be present in the here and now and not trapped in the past.

It is made using the alcohol method.

White Dead Nettle *(Lamium Album)*

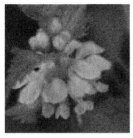

This essence is for removing the addictive effects of obsessive thought patterns.

White Dead Nettle is about addictions to objects, events or people. Sometimes animals get fixated on a toy, another animal and even meal times. The problem with that is that they will zone out of reality, to a point where they will not listen to their owner and may even stop eating. Addictions and obsessions are closely interrelated. White Dead Nettle helps your animal to detach themselves from emotional addiction or obsessions.

It is made using the alcohol method.

White Lotus *(Nyphaea Alba)*

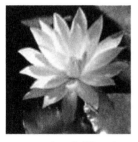

This essence is for bringing peace and unification to body, mind, spirit and soul.

White Lotus essence is about peace and tranquillity at all levels. Animals that pace or have stereotypical behaviour would benefit from taking this essence. This essence represents peace and will instil calmness and quietness within your animal. Tensions, fears, beliefs and opinions are all released so that they can just be. It can also act as an essence of purification by dissolving away things from their past that are no longer needed.

It is made using the alcohol method.

Wild Mallow *(Malva Sylvestris)*

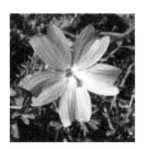

This essence is for helping to free us from energies that otherwise tend to possess us.

Wild Mallow brings hidden possessive energies to the surface where they can be dealt with. These are usually feelings caused by possessive owners. Wild Mallow will allow these feelings to be identified for what they really are, so their past will be seen for what it truly is and the power that their owner once held over the animal will be gone.

It is as if this essence tightens up the animal's feelings inside so that what is affecting them can be expelled. Rather like wringing out a cloth, the negative possessing energies are wrung out by Wild Mallow.

When your animal cannot see and yet instinctively knows that something is lurking in the shadows, this can cause your animal to feel spooked and unsettled.

It is made using the alcohol method.

Witch Hazel *(Hamamelis Mollis)*

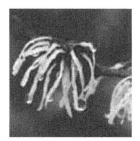

This essence is for those who sacrifice themselves in trying to live up to the expectations of others.

Witch Hazel is for those animals who are always trying to live up to the expectations of their owners or other people. They want to please and will look for continual approval. They may be continually under their owner's feet nipping at their heels, waiting in anticipation for acknowledgement. They feel that to let their owner down would be to fail and failure is never an option for an animal in a Witch Hazel state. They are often restless as they are very driven to find approval. This essence will allow your animal to let go of their neediness and to gain a wider view of the world around them.

It is made using the alcohol method.

Wood Anemone *(Anemone Nemorosa)*

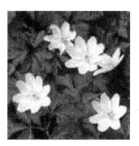

This essence is for use where there are very old difficulties – genetic or karmic.

The Wood Anemone is the essence for problems where the roots are very old, often before birth. Some of these may well be karmic. If your animal starts acting completely out of character this can be an indication of this state. Animals carry the genetic blueprint from their parents. If the mother was nervous, then they too would become nervous. There can be deep feelings of fear with the animal having no idea as to why they feel so fearful. Wood Anemone helps to clear these old blocked areas, illuminate them, and so resolve the issue. It is in the present, not in the past, that your animal must rebalance their life.

It is made using the alcohol method.

Yew (*Taxus Baccata*)

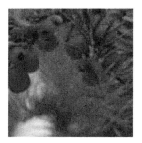

This essence is for resilience where previously the person has been too brittle – not bowing to the inevitable.

It is difficult to explain this essence in animal terms but it would be useful for animals who are very rigid in their attitude towards change.

Tensions make many people brittle and, although they may appear to be strong, they may suddenly crack under pressure. They are like cast iron which, although very strong, can fracture easily under a sudden shock.

They may have developed strong principles about which they are very protective. This can result in their reacting fiercely against what they see as opposing forces. Yew helps people to see that there is no sin in being both resilient and flexible, or indeed bowing before the storm. It also brings the discernment needed to assess accurately just what forces are involved in any particular situation. After all, only a fool will stand in the path of an express train!

Yew helps people to become less proud of their own ideas and concepts, more open to new approaches and ideas, and break up the rigidity of outmoded patterns of thought and behaviour. It is a very useful essence for people who have become trapped by their own beliefs and opinions.

It is made using the alcohol method.

Yorkshire Fog (*Holcus Lanatus*)

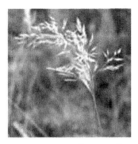

This essence is for grief, helping us to express it without becoming entangled in it.

Yorkshire Fog will enable your animal to open up to the pain of grief. Accepting hurt or grief is part of the healing process for your animal. It is a definite fact that animals grieve and need to process the loss of another animal or person. It is often very difficult for owners of animals to know whether their animal is grieving, as they don't wail or shed tears as a human would. Yorkshire Fog will help your animal to be open to grief, so they can express it more honestly.

It is made using the alcohol method.

Getting to Know the Bach Flower Essences

Dr Bach believed that the remedies were a 'God-sent gift to help heal our fears and anxieties; our mind being the most delicate and sensitive area of our body'. The remedies are therefore linked to our emotions. He listed them under seven headings. Arthur Bailey was asked by a client in Canada to produce the Bach Essences and to make them up in the exact same way as Dr Bach had nearly 100 years before.

Dr Edward Bach

The history begins nearly 100 years ago, with a man from Moseley, Birmingham, of Welsh origin. His name was Edward Bach (pronounced batch, as a lot of people could not say his name). He decided that he did not want to join his father's brass factory business but that he wanted to train as a doctor. He studied hard and got a job in London, working on Harley Street. It was around this time that the First World War started and he was keen to join. Unfortunately, he collapsed and was diagnosed with a tumour on his spleen. He was given just three months to live; it was at this point that I feel he did not want his life to be in vain. So he threw himself into his work, and before he knew it six months had passed.

Edward could reflect on how and why he had recovered from such a serious illness. He felt that it was due to his 'mind-set' that by having a positive view on life and not focussing on his illness, he could get well. This was the start of his study of personality traits in people and the start of his shift away from conventional medicine. He worked for several years in a homeopathic hospital and it was here that he created the homeopathic remedy 'nosodes'. He became very disillusioned with conventional medicine and began searching for an alternative.

He discovered that flowers had properties that could help people with emotional problems. By harnessing the flower energy, he could cure all kinds of personality traits. He worked for many years, covering various parts of the UK, to discover the 37 flower essences and one that is made of water. To find the correct flower he would often put himself in the emotional state he was looking to cure. At the end of his life he finally settled in Sotwell, Oxford. This is where the Bach Flower Centre is located, which continues to teach and educate people all about Bach flowers.

Edward died in 1936 at a young age of 50, just a few weeks after he had completed all his findings on the Bach flowers. It was almost as if his work was done, so he could finally let go and be. His legacy has grown and grown, with Bach flowers being sold in every part of the world. He was the start of the 'flower essence therapy' with many other pioneers discovering their own flower essence ranges, just like Arthur. These people were inspired by the brilliant work and research that Edward Bach did during his life time. In the last 50 years, they have been used extensively with animals, having a huge impact on their emotional well-being. It has raised many questions as to whether animals have 'souls', which we know they have; they walk a much more spiritual path than we do.

Remedies for Fear

Mimulus – *Fear of known things – your animal may feel shy or anxious.*
This bright yellow flower will give your animal true courage, when faced with a known fearful situation. As you can imagine, the world to an animal can often be filled with things that are fearful. If an animal is not socialised to as many things as possible when they are young, it can create a situation where your animal is literally scared of their own shadow. The vet, the postman, the dog next door and the wind whistling through the trees. The list is endless. Your animal may understandably be anxious but by giving this essence to them, you will be able to restore calmness and inner courage.

Cherry Plum – *Fear of losing your mind – your animal might lose control.*
It is one of the most useful essences to have; it has so many uses and animals seem to respond to it beautifully. Dr Bach said that this essence was for those who 'fear losing control'. The key phrase is 'losing control', which covers a multitude of possibilities: your animal bites, over-eats, cannot stop licking a sore spot until it bleeds, chases their tail for hours on end. Any situation where your animal is totally 'losing it', think Cherry Plum.

Aspen – *Fear of unknown things – your animal may feel anxious, but you don't know why.*
This essence's doctrine of signature perfectly describes its properties. If you look at the tree with its thin trunk supporting its sprawling branches, it shakes and quivers as the wind blows through its leaves. It is the tree that rattles at your window, giving you thoughts of nightmares as to the uncertainty of what this noise could be, leaving you with goose bumps and a pounding heart. Aspen is the essence for

fear with an unknown cause. It is excellent for nightmares; look for apprehension in your animal when there is no known cause.

Rock Rose – *Your animal feels extreme terror about something – inner panic, horror.*
This beautiful delicate yellow flower gives nothing away as to its purpose. It brings calm to animals who are suffering from extreme terror. They are so scared that their whole body shakes uncontrollably. Any conscious thought is disabled by this absolute terror. Their flight and fight response is often disabled to a point where they shut down. This is often caused by the lack of socialisation that they may have received when they were young, which means that they find the noises and goings-on in the world they live in very hard to deal with. This fear response can also be caused by abuse. An animal in a 'Rock Rose' state will greatly benefit from this essence.

Red Chestnut – *Your animal feels anxious about their loved ones.*
It is the most natural response for an animal to guard their young, as they are instinctively guarding the survival of their species. It is built into their innate behaviours so that the species can flourish. However, there are times when mothers become so protective of their young that they can be aggressive. This essence does not take away any motherly love, it just helps to put things in perspective so that the mother is less hostile and can enjoy her young as she was meant to.

Remedies for those who Suffer Uncertainty

Cerato – *Lack of trust in one's own decisions – your animal may seek advice from others.*
This beautiful flower is originally from Tibet and is the flower for wisdom. Sometimes we lose confidence in our own decisions and find confidence in what other people say. We end up on a path that is not our own destiny but that of others. The emotional traits associated with this essence may be difficult to see in your animal. It will help animals who are indecisive, or lack confidence with an urge to look for approval from their owners.

Scleranthus – *Your animal is unable to choose between two things – possible mood swings.*
I am not sure if it was by choice or is just coincidence but Dr Bach was very drawn to yellow flowers. This yellow common flower, up until recent years, grew in corn fields. Unfortunately, due to intensive farming it has now found a home in uncultivated ground and is less abundant. It is the remedy for uncertainty, where an animal is unable to choose. For example, where they want to sleep or what they want to eat. Scleranthus is the perfect remedy for travel sickness and mood swings. In fact, in any situation where there is huge imbalance.

Gentian – *Disappointment after a setback – your animal is easily discouraged.*
This beautiful purple flower is the perfect essence for any setbacks. Unfortunately, life is full of setbacks and this includes our animal friends too. The missed walk to the park, the owner going to work,

unscheduled box rest in a stable, etc. Don't get this essence confused with Gorse because on the scale of things, Gentian is for when our animals feel discouraged. By giving this essence we allow the animal to have their perseverance and drive restored, so they are all fired up to take on another day.

Gorse – *Hopelessness and despair – resignation, your animal is giving up.*
Dr Bach used to put himself into the exact state of the essence, so he understood exactly how it felt to be in that emotion. Some say that is what affected his life span, as he died a young man. The Gorse state is one of hopelessness and despair to a point where your animal just gives up; they stop eating and just wait for the end. Give your animal Gorse to bring back their hope; what may seem to be the end for them is purely a state of mind and can be remedied by taking this essence.

Hornbeam – *For procrastination – your animal cannot be bothered.*
Do you ever procrastinate, putting things off because the thought of doing something is just so overwhelming? Instead you let the housework pile up; "I will do it tomorrow," and tomorrow never comes. To label an animal to be in a Hornbeam state is difficult as they don't procrastinate or put things off. They have an innate survival code and putting things off could cost them their life. An animal in a Hornbeam state will probably look fatigued even when they have not done any exercise. They may be mentally unresponsive. If your animal looks like they cannot be bothered, think of Hornbeam as a ray of sunshine to bring back their oomph.

Wild Oat – *Uncertainty over direction in life – your animal has reached a crossroads.*
Like the oats that float from the plant on a windy day and scatter along the countryside paths and roads, the Wild Oat never settles. This essence helps those in life who too are drifting and never decide on their true path. It helps you to see your path more clearly. Animals have a very good sense of purpose but for those whose path is unclear, this is the essence for them. Animals become frustrated if there is a lack of uncertainty as to what they should do next.

Not Sufficient Interest in Present Circumstances

Clematis – *Your animal is a daydreamer – no great interest in life, in the present.*
This essence has been used with some success to help people with Alzheimer's. I have used it often with animals but it is important that you understand that you are not treating the condition, you are treating the individual animal. It helps the dazed emotions one may feel when they suffer from a shock. I call this the daydreamer essence, where we get caught up in our dreams. Dr Bach felt that it was very important that we all lived in the 'present'. Fantasying was another way that we are not connected to the 'here and now' as our dreams would never become a reality.

Honeysuckle – *Your animal is living in the past rather than the present.*
This truly wonderful flower essence has a multitude of uses. It is the essence for those who live in the nostalgic memories of the past. On a basic level, it may be because they feel that the past was much better than the present, often with rose tinted glasses. However, I have used this essence with an elderly patient suffering with dementia, trapped in a war memory of not being able to rescue children from a burning building. This beautiful remedy helped the person to leave that painful memory in the past, so she did not have to endure that nightmare again. Animals, too, that have suffered from abuse, feel that they cannot let that memory go. They cannot trust again, so it stops them from living in the present. This essence also works well for animals who suffer from separation anxiety; it allows them to understand that their owner will only be gone for a fleeting moment of time.

Wild Rose – *Apathy, your animal just cannot be bothered with life, resignation.*
This essence is often underrated and underused, yet its powers are quite profound. On the surface, it treats apathy and reassignment to the situation and the circumstances that an animal may find themselves in. They accept their conditions and don't hold out any hope for anything better. However, on a deeper level, this essence provides a ray of sunshine to those animals who are resigned to death. It is not the same as a Gorse state as their acceptance is that there is nothing better on the horizon.

Olive – *Exhaustion following mental or physical effort – your animal is tired.*
This is the only Bach essence which can be classed as helping a physical condition. It is for animals who are tired and exhausted after physical and mental work. It restores strength and energies, so they will be ready to take on another day of hard work.

White Chestnut – *Your animal cannot prevent thoughts – unable to settle.*
White Chestnut is often known as the sleeping essence and not because it makes you sleepy. What it does brilliantly is to stop all those thoughts rattling through your brain that keep you wide awake at night. They are reoccurring and will not switch off, causing you to toss and turn as the thoughts keep playing, like a broken record. In animals, they too are very unsettled, even though it is difficult to know what they are thinking. They will be pacing and may show stereotypical behaviour.

Mustard – *Your animal feels deep gloom or even despair for no reason, dark cloud descends.*
Dr Bach just could not get enough yellow flowers; it does seem to be the colour that dominates his essences. Again, this bright yellow flower has magic powers and helps to alleviate depression in your animal when there is no obvious reason. This foreboding feeling can be all-encompassing as it can trigger desperation in your animal. Just like the bright yellow sun that breaks up the dark clouds on a sunny day, lifting the gloom and despair, this essence too can offer happiness and joy to your animal.

Chestnut bud – *Your animal fails to learn from mistakes, failure to learn by experience.*
This essence is the perfect essence to give animals when they embark on any kind of training. It helps them to process the information so that new experiences do not become too overwhelming for them. When they keep making the same mistakes, it tends to knock their confidence. This essence will help them to make the right choices and to learn quickly.

Loneliness

Water Violet – *Your animal is aloof and wants to be on their own.*
The Water Violet likes to grow in solitary places, and this gives the clues as to the uses of this essence. A Water Violet type animal tends to be aloof and slightly detached from those around them. They feel happy in their own company but animals may also be in the Water Violet state when they are ill, choosing to find a quiet space. This essence is very useful now.

Impatiens – *Your animal is impatient and stressed.*
The doctrine of signature for this plant is one of impatience. Impatiens flower remedy treats impatience and irritability that is reflected in the shooting explosions of seeds from the plant, when the pod is ripe. This plant also grows rapidly compared to most plants. Animals that become impatient can become stressed and highly strung. They may be impatient to get out for their walk. They are always thinking of the next thing, so not savouring the exact moment. They may pull on their lead or get crotchety when their food is not on time. They may be unable to stand still.

Heather – *Your animal is self-centred, seeking company of anyone.*
I love this essence and it is because I often meet Heather type people. They are so full of their own needs that they cannot feel empathy for others. I suppose because I am a Centaury type, I listen to their never-ending stories about themselves, even when I may have somewhere important to be. A Heather trait in an animal can be easily seen in animals who are looking for attention, and that can be from anyone. They are literally in your face saying 'look at me, look at what I am doing. Listen to me, listen to how clever I am at barking'; sitting on your lap, following by your feet.

Over-Sensitivity to Influences and Ideas

Agrimony – *Your animal hides their worries, mental torture behind a cheerful face.*
One of the more difficult Bach Essences to identify in an animal. Why? Animals are open, they do not conceal their emotions like humans do. They are honest in how they feel. Yet! That does not mean they are not in an Agrimony state. They may be panting, showing signs of uneasiness; they are giving you signals and you just must listen to what they are saying. I have been able to use this essence with success, with an animal who was very quiet and subdued. The vet however recorded a very high blood pressure, which was very unusual for such a calm dog. On the surface, everything looked okay but clearly the little dog was hiding a multitude of problems.

Centaury – *Your animal is over-anxious and has the inability to say no.*
Doctrine of signature: the Centaury flower looks like the sun and follows the sun through the day. It opens and closes with the sun rise/ set. This shows an affinity to the heart. Dr Bach called those who were a Centaury type 'the salt of the earth'. Their kindness to serve, even when it does not benefit their own wellbeing, often means they are used as a door mat. Once walked over too many times, the mat shaken, they 'growl' then go back to their subservient ways. This essence will restore confidence in your animal with a certain swagger of assertiveness. Use this essence if your animal is showing submissive behaviour.

Walnut – *Protection from any change in life e.g. new home, new friend.*
The walnut with its hard exterior acts as protection from outside influences. This powerful essence can be used for a variety of situations, where change is involved. Change of owner, environment, food,

circumstance etc. It can be used where animals are going through a period of change, for example from puberty to adulthood. It also breaks links with the past so it is a wonderful remedy to use with rescue animals.

Holly – *Your animal is jealous and may hate.*
It is easy to see the doctrine of signature in this plant. It has prickly spikes that if they should catch your hand will make you bleed just like the colour of the berry and it hurts. Holly is the remedy for bitterness, jealousy, suspicion, spite and hatred. I don't think you can attribute these traits to an animal as they are very human emotions. However, when an animal is devoid of love in their life they can lash out, and they can be intolerant of new animal members to the household. When their heart is closed (often caused by animal abuse) it can be very difficult for them to love again.

For Despondency or Despair

Larch – *Your animal is lacking confidence, expecting failure.*
In life, we often miss out on adventure, as we are too scared to put ourselves out there, lacking confidence in our own ability, believing that we will fail. Animals too, for many reasons, can lack confidence, therefore need to be reassured. This is a great essence for rescue animals who have suffered from a knock to their confidence. Animals that have been convalescing, training, new owners and surroundings, etc. often need their vitality and belief to be restored. They may feel like a failure but when they take this essence they will feel like they can succeed in any area of their life.

Pine – *Your animal is feeling guilty even when it is not their fault. Do animals feel guilty?*
I am not sure if it is guilt, but I have seen my dogs, who usually bound down the stairs in the morning to be let out, sit quietly and wait until I have entered the kitchen, where I find the bin emptied all over the floor. I cannot say it is guilt but it is a definite knowing. Guilt is such a human emotion. How can we assume that an animal feels guilty? How can we measure this in our animals? This essence is for guilt whether it is by fault or caused by something out of one's control.

Elm – *For those who are usually confident – your animal is feeling overwhelmed.*
When you think of the Elm essence think of the word 'overwhelmed'. Animals lack confidence when faced with long term illnesses, training issues, new circumstances etc. They are usually confident but become worn down by being overburdened, which can make them feel inadequate. This essence restores competence and calmness.

Sweet Chestnut – *The anguish is so great – unbearable to carry for your animal.*

There are degrees of depression and this is the essence that treats animals who have come to a point emotionally where death is not an option. They have such a level of anguish that even death cannot take away the emotional pain. When you get to be in this emotional state everything has been tried. An animal self-mutilating is in a Sweet Chestnut state.

Star of Bethlehem – *Your animal is feeling grief, shock, bereavement, shock of a fall, accident, etc.*

This is probably one of the most famous Bach Flower Essences. It is the essence used most commonly in situations of grief and trauma, especially where there is shock. I would always consider this remedy when helping rescue animals. You can bet your bottom dollar that the animal has suffered from shock. It is a true story that Laurence Olivier purchased a bottle of Star of Bethlehem whenever he was on stage in London. He would down a whole bottle before his performance. It was most likely symbolic, as he would have only needed two drops from the bottle, which is the same as drinking the whole bottle. It is not the quantity that matters but the frequency.

Willow – *Your animal is feeling sorry for themselves – resentment, bitterness, self-pity, being treated unfairly by life.*

This is an easy remedy to remember, when you think of the term 'wallowing willow'. Blah, blah, blah, blah, bleating poor me, poor me, poor me. The animals caught up in this emotion feel desperately sorry for themselves and their life is full of woe. Of course, animals due to their survival skills are very rarely going to feel sorry for themselves. This is a luxury that humans alone seem to have bestowed upon themselves; they are experts at looking for sympathy. It is difficult to spot in animals, as they were put on this earth with more important things to do and a sense of feeling sorry for themselves is not always their highest priority.

Oak – *Your animal is exhausted but struggles on.*
The mighty oak tree stands proudly in the forest. Its strong leaf canopy protects the young saplings and animals below. Only after a storm has hit the forest and the mighty oak has fallen, laying bare its inner trunk, is the true devastation seen. The oak's centre is filled with decay, yet somehow it has stood strongly for years supporting the forest. An Oak animal will keep plodding on past exhaustion, taking little care of itself to a point that they will become ill. Their sense of duty is very strong and any illness or setback is classed as an inconvenience.

Crab apple – *Your animal is obsessed with uncleanliness.*
This essence is the perfect essence for repetitive behaviour such as stereotypical behaviour shown in animals. Box-weaving, excessive licking etc. Stereotypical behaviour is a way that an animal can release their stress by performing a ritual that serves no purpose. It is excellent for animals who have a flea infestation or similar and can be used as a detox after operations or vaccinations. See it as the cleansing essence.

Overcare for the Welfare of Others

Chicory – *Your animal loves you so much he/she will not leave your side and wants all your attention.*
The Chicory animal is always looking for attention, always under your feet; they are demanding and can be very yappy. The difference between Heather attention and Chicory attention is that a Heather animal looks for attention from anyone.

Vervain – *Your animal is FULL of enthusiasm and cannot settle.*
The Vervain state is one that is admirable as it echoes emotions of enthusiasm. When you are enthusiastic your spirits are very high but the down side is that you can get so caught up in this feeling that you can often miss what is going on in front of your very own eyes – although enthusiasm can have a very positive outcome. This essence is brilliant for animals who are SO enthusiastic it becomes SO overwhelming for owner and animal.

Vine – *Your animal is a bully.*
A good way to remember this remedy is to think of a bully. Animals naturally need a hierarchy structure, as this is what keeps the peace in the heard or the pack. A Vine type is when an animal is overbearing and is showing bullying traits to the other animals. They like to be in charge and like to dictate the rules, feeling that what they decide is the best course of action. (It is the opposite remedy to Centaury.)

Beech – *Your animal feels critical of or intolerant towards others/change.*
What did Dr Bach see in the Beech tree? It is a hardwood, yet it only has a shallow root system. It is a beautiful tree to look at and does have presence. In its essence form, it restores emotions of intolerance,

inflexibility and annoyance. Look for examples in your animal of inflexibility to change in diet, walks, location etc. Can your animal be bad-tempered? What do you think?

Rock Water – *Your animal is rigid and will not change.*
What led Dr Bach to discover the properties of Rock Water? Maybe it was his frequent walks in the countryside that helped him realise that if flowers have a unique energy, then so must everything else. Spiritual places have a unique energy, and this has already been harnessed by other Flower Essences producers. Rocks are rigid and inflexible and yet the water over a period softens the rocks. This essence is for those who set themselves punishing targets and will not stop until they have reached them. In animal terms, I would use this essence when the word 'inflexible' comes to mind. This essence should be used after Beech if your animal is still inflexible and intolerant of change.

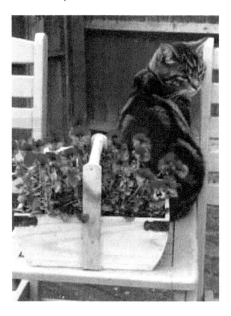

Getting to Know the Verbeia Essences

Heather

This is what the humans say: 'Increased energy, improved sleep, greater confidence. Helped me to refocus and make major life decisions.'

This is what the animals say: 'I now feel more attentive in my dog training lesson, I feel confident when I show jump, I coped well in my new home.'

Gorse

This is what the humans say: 'Calmness, relaxation. A more open approach to life. Patience came through appreciating the detail of life.'

This is what the animals say: 'I felt less stressed at the vets, I was able to wait good-naturedly for my food to be prepared, I have an overwhelming feeling of serenity, even when things seemed very worrying.'

Bracken

This is what the humans say: 'Cleansing and purifying. Stability and calmness but with a deep sort of exuberance from within.'

This is what the animals say: 'I felt unclean but now feel purified, I tended to obsess about things where I could not stop grooming, I feel that this obsession has now eased.'

Crowberry

This is what the humans say: 'Eased heaviness, lethargy, depression and a sense of unworthiness. Cleared the mind's fog, by helping to remove its cause. Seemed able to turn things round in an unexpected fashion.'

This is what the animals say: 'I was able to move forward after my owner was so sharp with me, I am able to see the world in a more positive way. I am happy in my new home, I feel like I have more energy.'

Winberry

This is what the humans say: 'Gave a sense of totality and wholeness. Helped with procrastination and difficulty in coming to the end of a project and making important changes in life, as another piece in the giant picture of life.'

This is what the animals say: 'I was lacking in enthusiasm when my owner wanted to play ball but now I am fully engaged in the game.'

Soft Rush

This is what the humans say: 'Created a nurturing supportive environment. Helped to address difficult issues from the past. Eased into stillness, quiet listening, remembering. Brought a sense of pure affection.'

This is what the animals say: 'I feel like I can cope now with my past abuse, I feel less stressed when I meet other animals or people.'

Fylfot

This is what the humans say: 'A sense of home. A sense of charity, sweetness and contentment. A very heart-centred gratitude and joy. A cornucopia of goodness.'

This is what the animals say: 'I feel safe, I feel grounded, I feel happy.'

Doctrine of Signatures

I speak about the doctrine of signatures quite often in my book and it is because I find the topic so interesting. Paracelsus was writing about this in the 1500s, long before Arthur had gone on his quest for flower essences. I am sure that Arthur understood that the colour, the smell, how it grows, where it grows, the time of year it grows, would give a good indication as to the healing properties it may have. Arthur writes about how the prickle of the holly leaf representing anger, and the shine of the holly leaf not allowing things to stick, represented being less sensitive to situations. The firethorn with its bright red berries is the perfect plant to balance excess 'fire energy'. The conifer mazegill, whose properties of the essence mirror the fungus itself, converts the dead wood of the past into new growth of a different form. I obviously do not know Arthur's thought process but I do know that he liked to communicate with the plants so he could understand the properties that they may have. He trusted his intuition but equally I feel that the plants were speaking to him through their form and how they grew on the deepest level possible. He chose his flowers by dowsing for them, but understanding what their healing properties are is a lot more complex. Maybe he was drawn again and again to the same tree or flower? Maybe he could read the doctrine of signatures and knew instantly what the flower essence was going to heal. The point here is that Arthur, deep down, understood the language of plants and made each essence individually per the need of the essence. For example, some are made in the sunlight, some in the moonlight and some have extra parts of the plant added such as the seeds.

How do the Bailey, Bach and Verbeia Essences Work?

I have a love and passion for working with flower essences as they are safe and very effective. Flower essences are vibrational medicines, which is based on the scientific principles that all matter vibrates to a precise frequency and when our bodies are out of kilter, they will vibrate at a lower frequency. Flower essences, therefore, will help to raise the lower frequency as their vibration is higher.

Vibrational medicine is a term used to describe therapies such as homeopathy, crystal healing, music therapy and colour therapy. What we cannot see does not mean that it does not exist. Almost everything around us has a living pulse inside of it, which vibrates at its own unique frequency. Vibrational medicines work on the principle that like attracts like and birds of a feather flock together. The higher frequency will therefore raise the lower frequency until they are both in harmony. The different parts of our physical, emotional, mental and spiritual entities resonate to various frequencies of vibration. If you think that your animal is made up of the energy of musical notes, if the notes are out of tune then your animal will be in disharmony. By taking flower essences, the out of tune song will be put back into a beautiful sounding melody; this will raise their spirits. Have you ever listened to uplifting music, which makes you feel alive, happy and invigorated? This is how flower essences work – they will drag your animal away from their woes, their fears and grief.

Disharmony shows in the energy field before it manifests in the physical body.

Animals suffer from the same emotional problems as people. They grieve, they get depressed, they feel stressed. These cause imbalances, which if detected using science can be seen in the animal's aura. If this is not addressed and the animal suffers grief caused by the loss of a loved one, theoretically he/she may go on to develop for example a heart problem, tumour etc. All bad emotional problems vibrate at a lower frequency and each emotion vibrates at its own unique frequency. By using flower essences to address the emotional problem, it raises the vibration to treat the grief so the disease can be avoided altogether. If the grief is never addressed and the tumour removed, it will possibly grow back.

The highest frequency emotion is enthusiasm; love and joy also fall into this category. This is followed by pain (emotional or physical) which is followed by anger. The next lower frequency emotion is fear, which is followed by grief. Below grief is apathy. Finally, the lowest frequency emotion is unconsciousness (meaning it is so awful we have completely blocked out those situations from our lives). It makes sense that the happiest experiences would reap the highest frequencies. Who would not want to be happy all the time? When you make up a flower essence treatment bottle, you are in fact making up a magical melody to heal their woes.

Flower essences work beautifully with animals as they do not carry the baggage of life like we do. They deserve the chance to heal from any sensitive problem, so they can happily move forward with their life.

The do's and don'ts of taking the Bailey, Bach and Verbeia Essences

Are Bailey, Bach and Verbeia Essences Safe?

In over 100 years of use there has not been a single adverse reaction recorded. Bailey, Bach and Verbeia Essences are hypoallergenic and drug free. They contain the 'energy' of the plant and contain no components of the plant, so there is no potential for toxicity. This means that there is no way you can cause harm to your animal. They are 100% safe and work to raise the 'vibrational energy' of your animal. They will help your animal to feel less stressed, less anxious and more at peace.

Can Bailey, Bach and Verbeia Essence Help Physical Problems?

They cannot directly help your animal's physical problem, but they can help with the way your animal deals with their physical problem. The 'key' here is to understand that each animal will react in a different way 'emotionally' to the same physical problem. It is important to understand that you are not treating the physical illness directly, you are treating your animal individually for how they are dealing with their physical illness. By changing your animal's outlook, it will have positive effects on their physical condition.

Every animal has their own personality, which is unique to them. Some will mope and sulk feeling sorry for themselves, needing an essence for despondency and self-pity. Other animals will be positive and carry on as if nothing has happened. They will need an essence for reflection and understanding. The point is that the same physical illness manifests but the emotional coping mechanisms will be different. Animals have countless emotional feelings that are as unique and complex as those seen in humans. If we pigeonhole a dog as a dog and a cat as a cat, and never look past the stereotype of their species, we will miss the beautiful array of emotional messages that they are showing us daily.

Case Study 1

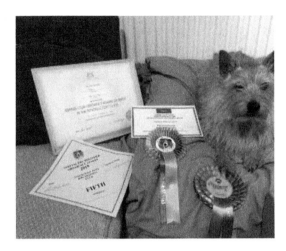

Cassie is an elderly dog, and is a dog I have been working with for many years. Initially when she first came to me, she was lacking in confidence and was feeling generally fed up. I made up a treatment bottle of Bailey, Bach and Verbeia Flower Essences for her with the following essences listed below.

Walnut – Difficult transition from puppyhood
Lilac – Personal development stunted
Scabious – Initiates healing
Sumach – Fear to accept her own gifts
Fylfot – To help her feel safe

Cassie had a remarkable change from taking the essences. She grew in confidence and as in her photo above entered many obedience competitions and won them. She went on to a photo shoot to London and her energy and love of life increased. Her owner said that even her hearing and eyesight improved. This beautiful little dog had got her 'mojo' back and was loving every single second of it. The other interesting thing that happened was that her brother had taken some of the essence that had been put in a water bowl and he too started to win competitions.

More proof that putting the essences in a water bowl that other animals have access to shows that they too need one or more of the ingredients.

How do I Choose the Correct Bailey, Bach and Verbeia Essence For My Animal?

In a lot of situations, you will know exactly why your animal is behaving in a certain way. This will make your choice of essence a whole lot easier than when you have no clue as to the new behaviour your animal is exhibiting. When this happens to me, I take a piece of paper and record all the things I can think of that may have caused stress to my animal. I list their behaviour, any physical problems, their history and any key words to help me understand what is truly going on. What you then have is a complete picture of all the elements in your animal's life. From this list, you can match a flower essence to the behaviour.

I have created a form to make things easier for you. As we are unable to be with our animals all of the time, there will be things in their lives that cause them stress and we will be totally unaware; in other words, we are clueless.

How to use the Bailey, Bach and Verbeia Form

I have designed the following form so you can use it to brainstorm your thought process. When you are faced with an animal problem, you can often not see the wood for the trees. There may be so much going on that it is often difficult to get to the root of the problem. You will also see that the owner, too, is having an impact on the emotional well-being of their animal.

Behaviour
This can cover a multitude of situations: barking, excessive licking, aggression, fear, excitement etc.

Physical
How does the animal look? What condition is their fur, their hooves, their nails? How do their eyes look? Are they thin or fat?

History
The more you know of it, the better.

Learnt Behaviour
Do they bark to get you to take them for a walk?

Welfare
Have they been rescued?

Key Words
Pacing, hiding, fearful, uncertain

Client
Intense, not listening, stressed, lacking confidence

Behaviour	Physical	History		Remedies
Learnt	Welfare	Other	Key words	Client

You can also dowse for the correct flower essence, which was Arthur's preferred choice.

How to use a Pendulum

Using a pendulum will allow you to not only choose the correct flower essence for your animal, but it will allow you to find out what is going on with your animal at a deeper level. Learning how to use a pendulum correctly will help both you and your animal to make the right choice.

For example, it will help you to choose the correct flower essence, food, the correct vet and everything else in your animal's life with a 'yes' or 'no' answer. The correct term for using a pendulum is called 'dowsing'. I will be honest and say that no one really knows how a pendulum works.

- Purchase a pendulum that you feel drawn to.
- Spend a few moments in a quiet, relaxing state.
- Hold the top of the chain in your dominant hand and ask the pendulum: show me 'yes'. Wait for a response, as your pendulum will swing in a certain way unique to you. This will always be your 'yes' answer from now on.
- Again, hold the top of the chain and ask the pendulum: show me 'no'. Wait for a response. Again, your pendulum will swing in another unique way, which will always be your 'no' answer from now on.
- From the previous list of Bailey, Bach and Verbeia Essences in alphabetical order: point your non-dominant hand at each essence name and ask: "Does (name of your pet) need this essence at this exact moment in time?" With your dominant hand holding the pendulum, wait for a yes or no answer. Write down any yes responses on a piece of paper. These will be the Bailey, Bach and Verbeia Flower Essences that your pet will need.

There are other fun ways in which your animal will take control of their own healing. Randomly flick through the Bailey Handbook, think of the issue, close your eyes and stop at a page where you feel you should stop. This will be the flower essence that they need. Show the bottles to your animal, they will show interest in the bottle they require.

You can also let your animal smell each bottle; to us it will smell of vodka, but our animals are clever peeps and they will be able to pick up on the 'vibrational' energy of each bottle.

You can also cut out photographs of the flowers and place them around the floor. Your animal will naturally gravitate towards the picture of the flower that they require. Animals are far more sensitive to energies than we are and just because it is a picture of the flower, it too will have its own vibrational energy which your animal will be able to pick up on. It is proven that some animals can sense chemical changes in groundwater that occur when an earthquake is about to strike. They can read the signs long before the earthquake erupts, which shows why they are equally as sensitive to vibrational medicine.

What Should I use to Dilute my Essences?

This may sound like a strange question, but it is one that needs careful thought. The energy of the flower needs to have a perfect place to store their magical energy. Did you know that we are made up of 60% water and over 60% of the earth is covered in water? It therefore makes total sense to me that water would be the best vehicle to store the magic of the Bailey, Bach and Verbeia Flower Essences. Without water, all living things would die.

There have been studies performed by a Professor Emoto, who proved that the power of words had a huge impact on the way the crystals formed in the water as they began to freeze. Water that had been shouted at formed into disjointed crystals, whereas water that had been spoken to lovingly or prayed with formed into beautiful stunning crystals. Just think that here in the UK, every glass of water from the tap has at some stage passed through someone else! Who knows if that person was happy or sad? The energy of that person is stored as a memory in the water, which eventually we drink. What effect is that having on us, do you think? Bailey, Bach and Verbeia Flower Essences need to be stored in a water that is as pure as possible. This is so that the flower essence can work its beautiful magic in the most vibrant way possible.

Water which is Good for Flower Essences

Mains water that has been purified through a filter and then boiled and cooled is recommended. The boiling helps it lose any stored information.
- Glass bottle mineral water with a mineral content of less than 200mg/litre.

Not Good for Flower Essences

- Mineral-rich spring or mains water with a mineral content of 1000mg/litre or more.
- Water contained in plastic bottles can be contaminated by the plastic leaking into the water, so is not recommended.
- Tap water which has not been boiled.

- Unfiltered water, which is pumped through the water system under pressure, which makes it less able to hold on to information.

How do I make up a Treatment Bottle?

You will need the following:
- 30ml Treatment Bottle
- Chosen Flower Essences
- Label
- Still Mineral Water
- Pen

Armed with the flower essences, which have been chosen by either you or your animal, you will need to make up a treatment bottle. You can put up to seven flower essences in each bottle, but if possible try to keep the choice to a maximum of three. This is my opinion, but I truly feel that 'less is more'. It allows you to focus on the main issues of your animal's behaviour. When seven flower essences are added, the issues can become clouded; and again, my opinion, but I feel that the treatment bottle will not be as effective, as there will be too many 'vibrational' flower energies.

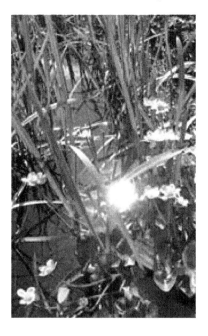

- Add **two** drops from each flower essence to the treatment bottle.
- Fill the treatment bottle with still mineral water.
- Label the treatment bottle with the animal's name, flower essences, dosage and date.
- Shake the treatment bottle vigorously to release the flower energies; also shake each **time** you use the treatment bottle.
- Give four drops four times a day.
- **This treatment bottle will keep for three weeks in the fridge.**

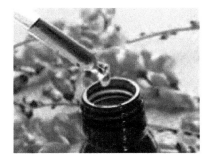

The four drops can be added to your animal's food, drinking water, treats and licked from your hand; in fact, any ingenious way you can think of.

Never insert the pipette of the treatment bottle into your animal's mouth as it can break off and hurt your animal. It would also become contaminated, making the treatment bottle useless.

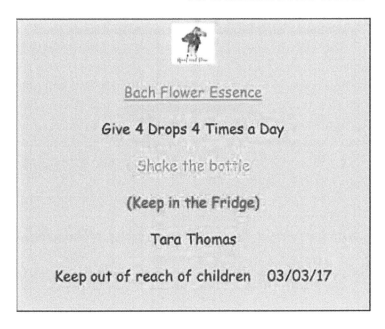

Bach Flower Essence

Give 4 Drops 4 Times a Day

Shake the bottle

(Keep in the Fridge)

Tara Thomas

Keep out of reach of children   03/03/17

If you **do not have** a treatment bottle you can add 'two' drops of your chosen flower essence from the stock bottle to your animal's drinking water. Each time they drink they will get a 'dose' of the flower essence. If you are adding the flower essence stock bottle to drinking water for a horse, I would personally add ten drops as the volume of water in a bucket is much more than a bowl. Fish **cannot** have flower essences added to their water directly; but by placing the treatment bottle next to the fish tank, shake the bottle vigorously every day, so the 'vital life force energy' is released.

If you would like to use the Bailey, Bach or Verbeia Flower Essences externally, make up a mist bottle.

You will need:
- A mist bottle
- Chosen flower essence
- Still mineral water
- Label
- Pen

Mist bottles can be used to spray into an area such a stable, kennels, and any room. A mist bottle is excellent for dogs or cats who suffer from travel sickness, as it can be sprayed into the car before they get into it. Also, spray the mist bottle into a horse trailer before the horse enters. They can also be sprayed onto the animal's fur or feathers. Some birds enjoy having their feathers misted; but if they do not, spray the mist bottle into the cage when the bird is not in there. Always make sure that you write the date on the bottle on the day it is made up, so you will know when it has gone out of date and then will be able to make up a fresh supply.

- Add two drops of your chosen flower essences into the mist bottle.
- Fill with still mineral water. Label the mist bottle with the animal's name, flower essences and date.
- Shake the mist bottle vigorously to release the flower energies; also, shake each **time** you use the mist bottle.
- **This mist bottle will keep for three weeks in the fridge.**

How Long do I Give Bailey, Bach and Verbeia Essences for?

- For long-term or chronic issues, give four times daily.
- For acute issues, give four times a day **up to** as often as every few minutes.

The beauty of Bailey, Bach and Verbeia Essences is that you **can do no harm**, so you do not need to worry about giving your animal too many doses as the treatment bottle only contains the energy of the flower essences. Remember also that frequency is more important than quantity.

Keep an eye on any behavioural changes; some animals respond immediately, and others will take a few weeks to respond to the essences. Write down any changes that take place, as it will help confirm that you have made the correct Bailey, Bach and Verbeia essence choice. If there is no change within a couple of weeks, you will need to rethink your choices and consider again what is really going on with your animal.

Is it Harmful for my Other Pets to Drink Water that Contains Bailey Essences?

This is a question that I am asked often, so I will answer it as best I can. As Bailey, Bach and Verbeia Essences contain only the 'energy' of the flowers they contain **no** component of the flower; therefore, they have no harmful side effects. Essences that are not needed by an animal will have no effect. However, there are times where the other animals will benefit, as unbeknown to you they may require a particular flower essence. It has happened often that other animals in the family, who initially were thought to not have any problems, will too change their behaviour in a positive way.

It is often only at the time of crisis that owners will turn to Bailey, Bach and Verbeia Flower Essences, when in actual fact if we turned to them sooner our animals would be mentally and emotionally so much better. Stress within our animals is on the increase and as owners we need to be more responsible and to try to understand what our animal needs.
• Understand your animal and their species
• Make sure your animal is socialised from an early age
• Meet the needs of your animal e.g. exercise
• Do not overfeed
• Feed the correct diet to your animal
• Do not over-vaccinate (personal view)
• Have the correct fittings such as in saddles and collars to prevent low-level pain.
• Never diagnose your animal, always take your animal to a vet if unsure.

How to Amplify the Bailey Essences

I have found that you can use a copper pyramid to enhance the 'life force energy' of the Bailey, Bach and Verbeia Essences. The shape of a pyramid allows it to collect energy, just like a solar panel would. Copper is an excellent conductor of energies and the pyramids are also natural ionisers and help to improve air quality. How they work is to do with the shape of the pyramid and the way energy is stored in the the vortex centre. Items placed at the centre will absorb this energy until they are fully regenerated. The position of the pyramid is also an important factor – with a four-sided pyramid, if one of the pyramid sides should face true north, the energies within the pyramid are much stronger. When I started to use a copper pyramid I noticed that the treatment bottles were more effective when used with my animal clients.

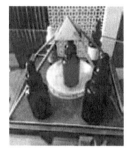
Stock bottles and treatment bottles should be placed under the pyramid for up to two hours. If you want the strongest life force energy, then place the bottle under the pyramid during the morning. It is very important to keep your pyramid dust free, as this will affect the energy. If using more than one bottle, do not allow it to touch another bottle.

The Magic of Bailey, Bach and Verbeia Flower Essences

With over 14 years of experience of working with flower essences and animals, an unusual thing started to happen. Whilst making up the essences for an animal, the animal would become calmer even though they had not taken the essences. It made me re-evaluate flower essences with a different understanding of how flower essences work.

Take a moment to let go of your preconceptions of the Bailey, Bach and Verbeia Flower Essences; don't be trapped by the confines of your own mental state of understanding. If we take the stance that we are all 'one' then there is no me and no you, there can only be unity and oneness. If a scientist puts a flower essence under the microscope and methodically tested it, they would only find traces of alcohol and, of course, the water that carries the energy. So where is that flower energy? You cannot see it, you cannot measure it, yet the 'life force' energy it has is so vibrant and healing. With the concept of 'oneness' you are able to treat an animal on the other side of the world without actually giving the animal any contents of the treatment bottle. This has happened to me on so many occasions now that I make a point to connect to the energy of the animal I am working with while I make up the treatment bottle.

Make up the treatment bottle in the same way you usually would, take a picture of the animal that you are treating and hold the intention that you are offering the remedy to the animal. In this powerful intention, the 'life force' energy can connect to the animal. If you understand what this 'oneness space' means, you will know that there is no distance or time. By placing the flower remedy over the picture and ideally a piece of hair (called a witness of the animal), the animal is indeed receiving the 'life force' energy of the flowers. You can even create a little flower essence shrine, with the photo and the treatment bottle. Keep the shrine clean and dust-free. Shake the bottle and offer, with intention to the animal, the flower essence morning and night. There is no need to decant any drops from the bottle, as it is the energy that is inside the bottle that is working its magic.

I truly believe that once an animal knows that you are trying to help them, they can connect to the energy of the flowers even if they live thousands of miles away. There is no issue with distance or time as 'flower energy' has no constraints to keep it trapped within our own concepts of these rules.

Case Study 2

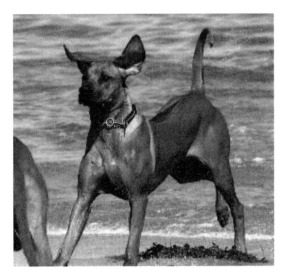

The interesting thing about this case is that Otis's behaviour began to change as soon as I dowsed for his essences. Without even taking them, he was able to work with the 'life force energy' of the flowers. Otis had been quite dominant over the other dogs in his household and would run at full pelt and barge into them. He was very unsettled when his owner left and would often chew holes in the furniture.

Flower essence report given to his owner:

Chosen by Otis using dowsing.

Betony

Otis is showing that he has hidden fears; he may not truly understand what he is fearful of. It could be something that derived from puppyhood and is probably something that you are not even aware of. Betony will help him to make sense of what is going on and it will help him to move forward.

Black Locust

Otis is showing that he is feeling nervous and this uncertainty is making him feel nervous. He may be picking up on other energies which he is trying to quantify. For some reason, he is feeling vulnerable and this undefined feeling is making him feel defenceless.

Deep Red Peony

It will bring light to Otis's worries, which will work hand-in-hand with the first two essences. It has been used with children who have attention deficit and hyperactivity syndrome. It is for those who see the world as a frightening place and feel disempowered and alone. I truly feel, by the choice that Otis has made, there is something unnerving him and he does not know how to make sense of it. Deep Red Peony is the key to unlocking his worries.

Dog Rose

We want to offer comfort and support to Otis, as he starts to see things clearly. It will offer support if things get difficult. It offers loving protection and will offer Otis immediate relief from any uncertainty.

Holly Leaf

Otis is feeling pent up; it is difficult to say that it is anger, but it could be frustration. There are two forms of anger; the first is a natural reaction to unreasonable provocation. However, if for any reason Otis is unable to deal with this frustration as it arises, it will be held within the mind and the body and can emerge as resentment. It is the retained anger that will cause difficulties for Otis. Holly Leaf will help Otis by offering him a breathing space to let go of his frustration. It will also take the 'sting' out of the situation by deflecting any intended desire to 'hurt' another other dog.

The thing about Otis was that the problem was not as it seemed, even when taking the flower essences. Otis not only quieted down a small bit, but what unfolded was profound.

Feedback

He does seem to be calming down a little (though whether that's due to us being at home constantly over Christmas, which means he's more active/not anxious I'm not sure); however, his obsession with Maali's urine and his licking of his willy still continues the same as it always has. The conclusion I'm coming to is that we are trying to correct a 'behaviour' when in actual fact it's just his personality and he will grow out of it as he matures. You have been wonderful in your quest to find an essence that would hit the jackpot.

Thank you so, SO much for everything you have done and I wish you a very happy and healthy New Year.

The point is that sometimes we are looking at behaviours as if there is something wrong. When Otis's owner actually listened to him, she realised that this was his natural playful personality. Sometimes we are trying to 'fix' things that are not actually broken. When we take the time to actually listen to our animals, we are often amazed at what they have to say.

Otis is a dog that I worked with again two years later, after he lost two dogs within the household in a very short amount of time. I have discussed this case in detail further on in this book.

Can Bailey, Bach and Verbeia Essences be Used with Medicine from a Veterinarian or Other Treatments?

Bailey, Bach and Verbeia essences are truly 'perfect' to complement any medicine from your vet. They **cannot** interact with Western medicine because they contain only the 'energy' of the flower. They can be added to creams, mixtures, compresses and any washes.

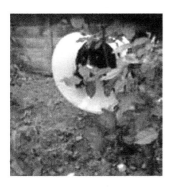

*Bailey, Bach and Verbeia essences can be used alongside or combined with any other healing therapy with **no** adverse problems. If your animal is being treated by a Flower Essence Practitioner, then they will need to let the vet know that your animal is taking the essences. This is good practice and it is the law of the land as your vet always remains responsible for the health and welfare of your animal. If you are treating the animal yourself then there is no legal requirement for you to let them know, but it makes sense that your vet is aware of any treatment that your animal is receiving.*

Healing Crisis

Although very rare, sometimes the Bailey, Bach and Verbeia Essences can seemingly exacerbate the condition that you are trying to heal. For example, your animal may become more fearful for a few days. This is because the essences are cleansing your animal's emotions, which may have been ingrained within your animal for a very long time. When strong emotions or repressed abuse issues are finally allowed to surface, they may surface very quickly. How your animal copes with a healing crisis will be dependent on how painful these emotions really are. You can look at it in two ways: The first being that your animal is finally letting go a very painful memory, and second that they are enlightened to that memory. The healing crisis could also manifest as a physical symptom such as diarrhoea, a rash or even a cough. You should always get your animal checked out by a vet to make sure that it is not something else. If the healing crisis is severe, I would suggest reducing the doses of the essences and to also use other Bailey, Bach and Verbeia Essences to support the changes that are happening. During this time, you will need to give your animal plenty of water and allow them to have as much rest as possible. Give your animal lots of cuddles and be very supportive during this time. They may even have an energy boost, which is not uncommon after a healing crisis. Do not put your animal under any stress and know that this is a very short-lived process.

Through my research and trials, I now believe that animals know best in how to treat themselves. I believe in self-medication; this is done by putting the essence in a separate water bowl so that they are not forced to take the essence more than they need in their normal daily water intake. In this way, they decide the dosage and when they no longer need to medicate. I wonder if this will lead to a lower frequency of animals in crisis, or maybe completely eradicate crisis in healing whereby we have to intervene and reduce or stop the dosage for them.

The Bailey, Bach and Verbeia Trials

I was asked in May 2016 by Bailey Essences to create a range of essences for animals. It was an honour and a wonderful project to head. Over the summer, I meditated with the essences and I asked Arthur Bailey to help me with their creation. It was a beautiful summer as there were so many long sunny days. I would sit outside in my garden, with the sun on my back and draw inspiration from the flowers in my garden. Over that summer, I created seven composite essences for our wonderful animal friends. I drew motivation from the knowledge of the animals that I had worked with over the last 14 years, those who had been emotionally damaged by abuse and neglect. It was here that flower essences had given them hope. The first thing I did was to decide on the range of emotions that I wanted the composites to treat. What was troubling our animals emotionally? How could my range have the most impact? And who would help me test the range? My Hoof and Paw Academy had been up and running for some time. I asked the group if anyone could help me to run the trials. I was blessed with an astounding response. These amazing women gave their time selflessly and each connected with the animals and owners in their own special unique way.

1. **Space/fear aggression (me)**
2. **Socialisation (Mandy Johnson)**
3. **Liberation (Emma Salt)**
4. **Separation (Denise Marsden)**
5. **Grief (Paula Ferrant)**
6. **Fears (Mandie Danks)**
7. **Transition (Fiona MacKay)**

The first thing that I needed to do was to meet up with Mandy and Paula, so that we could come up with a plan of action. Mandy designed the feedback forms and we discussed what type of information we needed, such as vet permission, description of the problem, a list of animal behaviours and so much more. I put out an advert on my Hoof and Paw Facebook page and was overwhelmed by the amount of interest and the commitment of people who wanted to trial one of the composite essences. This was further proof that animals were suffering emotionally. Each animal was then categorised as to which trial they would be in and the coordinator of the trial then contacted the owner and it was here that relationships started to be formed. The three of us met often and during one of those meetings we made up the seven composite essences, asked for Arthur Bailey's inspiration and created a spiritual environment of love and positivity. Each composite was carefully packaged with instructions, stock bottle and treatment bottle and then posted to locations dotted all over the world. The trials lasted for 12 weeks and it was a huge success. The data is still being processed and we hope to produce a scientific paper. Please use this link which will be used to show our findings. *https://caroline382.wixsite.com/mysite*

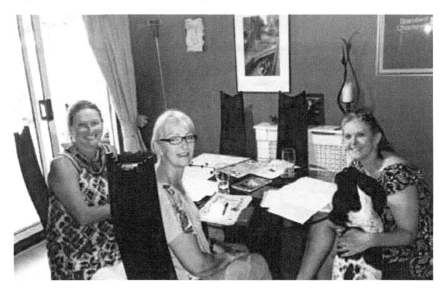

The Purpose of the Seven Animal Composite Essences

1. Space/Fear Aggression

The Space/ Fear Aggression Essence has been created for animals that like to protect their own space. This could be due to your animal feeling unsettled when another animal enters their aura, forcing them to lash out aggressively. The aggression can equally be caused by fear as your animal learns that by lashing out first, they will then keep the other animal at bay. If the aggression is not addressed it can escalate and become out of control; I strongly suggest that they wear a muzzle. This is to protect the other dog/s and your dog from being hurt. The definition of aggression is the threat of harm from another individual involving snarling, growling, snapping, biting, barking, and/or lunging. A side effect of this essence is that it supports dogs who bark excessively. The Space/Fear Essence is made from a blend of Bailey, Bach and Verbeia Flower Essences. It contains flower essences such as Cherry Plum and Vine and others to support the change desperately needed to restore balance.

2. The Socialisation Essence

This essence has been created to affectionately support animals who have not been socialised to the world they live in. This is often the case when animals have been taken away from their mothers and siblings too early. It is a modern misconception that eight weeks is the optimal time for a kitten or puppy to leave their home. This is a crucial socialisation period when animals learn from their mother and family about how to be a cat or a dog. If this window of learning is disrupted and your animal has not experienced the right experiences, what you will have is an animal that may exhibit certain fearful behaviours such as fear, aggression, uncertainty, lack of confidence, and they may lack communication skills when conversing with other animals. A side effect of this essence is that it can help to shift a memory developed out of a trauma that is still present in the psyche many years later. The Socialisation Essence is made from a blend of Bailey, Bach and Verbeia Flower Essences. It contains flower essences such as Rock Rose and Lily of the Valley and others to support the change needed to become confident and certain of their environment.

3. The Liberation Essence

The Liberation Essence has been created to support your animal as he/she moves from the Rescue Centre into their new home. This is a critical time for animals as they settle into their 'forever' home. If you have an animal that has been abused, it will often mean that they will certainly come with a lot of baggage. This will often affect how long it takes for them to settle into their new home. They will frequently suffer from trust issues, fear issues, anxiety issues and toilet problems, and will often form an unhealthy bond with their liberator which can lead to separation anxiety. Your animal can be supported emotionally by taking this combination essence, as it will allow them to accept the past by healing their psychological wounds. When your animal accepts the past, they will certainly be able to embrace the future and their new life. The Liberation Essence combination is made from a balance of Bailey, Bach and Verbeia Flower Essences. It contains flower essences such as Leopardsbane, Soft Rush and others to support change for a better future.

4. The Separation Anxiety Essence

The reason the Separation Anxiety Essence has been created is because this is now such a growing problem and if not treated it can result in the deterioration of your dog's mental and physical health. Dogs have evolved from wolves where pack mentality is instinctive. The most natural thing for them is to hang out with you all day. Unfortunately, with bills to pay this is not always possible. If your dog has not learnt the coping skills of how to be alone, they can become very distressed and exhibit behaviours such as barking, whining, howling and even destroying furniture. This Combination essence has been designed to support change while a behavioural plan is put in place. (This must be from a reputable behaviourist or if you are to do this yourself, you must make sure that you understand the whole process completely.) The Separation Anxiety Essence combination is made from a blend of Bailey, Bach and Verbeia Flower Essences. It contains flower essences such as Sea Campion and Honeysuckle along with others. These will support your dog as he/she learns that being 'home alone' is not so bad.

5. The Grief Essence

The grief essence has been created to support animals who have experienced loss. This could be the loss of their owner, their animal companion or even the loss of something physical like their favourite toy. This combination essence is made from a synergy of Bailey, Bach and Verbeia Flower Essences. Grief can be defined as a very deep sadness and it is a normal reaction to loss or change. Animals, just like their human owners, will grieve and will often exhibit behaviours to show that they too feel loss. They sometimes go off their food, look depressed and can become withdrawn. They may pine, circle and even show OCD behaviours such as excessive licking. This combination essence contains flowers such as Star of Bethlehem and Trailing St John's Wort. These essences with others, too, make sure that the grief is being freely expressed by your animal so that it does not get locked inside of them. Just remember that grief is a natural process and will eventually pass in time. This Combination essence will beautifully support that journey and it is recommended that if you too are grieving, you should take the essence along with your animal.

6. The Fear Essence

This Fear Essence has been lovingly created to support animals who are in a state of fear when faced with a situation that they are terrified of. This could be the vet, fireworks, postman, groomer, the car, plastic bag, farrier and anything else that instils fear within your animal. The reasons might be unknown to even the animal but the behaviours exhibited are usually the same: shaking, panting and hiding. The definition of 'fear' is that of an unpleasant emotion caused by the threat of danger, pain, or harm. Whether the threat is real or imagined, the feeling or condition of feeling fear will still be the same. Fear will often trigger the flight and fight response and if your animal is not able to act this out, as nature has intended, there will be a continual release of hormones which will have nowhere to go. This will then have a knock-on effect on your animal's health in other ways. The Fear Essence is made from a blend of Bailey, Bach and Verbeia Flower Essences. It contains flower essences such as Aspen and Bracken and others to support the change needed so that courage can blossom, just as any beautiful flower would.

7. The Transition Essence

Transition is a combination of essences made from the Bailey, Bach and Verbeia Flower Essences. It is made with the intention of helping your animal move though any type of transition. It has been created to help animals who are terminal or at end of life. It has **not** been created to speed up the end of life process, but to address any fears that they may have. It has been created so it can offer peace when 'fear' is abounding. It contains flower essences to support change such as Bistort and Walnut; but also, flowers to support fears caused by the unknown, such as Aspen. It will help your animal to come to terms with their illness so they can deal with it daily. This essence will help your animal cope with the stages before death. It offers tranquility and serenity, but most of all dignity. It is recommended that the owner also take the essence at the same time as the animal. The word transition means 'change' therefore the 'Transition essence' can be used to help any animal through any key changes in their life.

As with any trial that is run correctly, there were a few anomalies where the composite essence did not have the desired effect that it was supposed to have. I contacted the owners of the animals and arranged a consultation via Skype. It became clear to me that – although the animals had initially presented with problems that looked like the same behaviour as, for example, those that the space/fear aggression essence was created to treat – after further investigation, the root of the problem was very different to what the composite essence had been designed to do. In all cases I made up a bespoke remedy and this alleviated the problem. Animals are all unique, and we should understand that to treat the behaviours we need to first understand the root of what drives these behaviours.

Self-Selection of Bailey, Bach and Verbeia Flower Essences

The invaluable evidence gained by running such a big trial also uncovered other behaviours which allowed me to experiment in more detail. Self-selection of flower essences started to become more noticeable from the feedback that I was receiving. I also decided to teach self-selection as part of my Hoof and Paw Practitioner Course Curriculum. It seemed that even though the bottles looked the same and smelt the same, animals could pick up on the different energy that each bottled contained. So instead of teaching to put two drops of each essence in a treatment bottle, I started to teach to put two drops of essence into separate bowls of water and let the animal choose. This is revolutionary in giving control back to the animal and respecting their freedom to choose. Let's stop 'doing to' the animal and let's start listening to our animals, as you know what, they really do know what is best for themselves. Let's let go of the ego that we know best and swallow a spoonful of humility and graciousness, that maybe there is much more to learn.

The coursework that I received back from my students more than confirmed this theory. By allowing animals to oversee their own healing, more shifts from bad behaviour to good behaviour became evident. This is an area of research that I will be continuing to explore in the future with the help of my students. Here is a link of my own dog Lenny using self-selection to choose the perfect Verbeia Flower Essence just for himself.

https://www.youtube.com/watch?v=Mok1pqbFGjU

It clearly shows that his choice was not a coincidence but a deliberate act of 'this is what I want'.

The Mirroring Effect of Bailey Bach and Verbeia Flower Essences

What do you think of when you think of a mirror? I immediately think of the mirror from the Harry Potter books – the Mirror of Erised, which reflected what Harry most desired in life: to see his parents again. What a powerful gift that would be; but a mirror reflects the perfect image of the person or animal, every line, expression, feather or hoof.

Through my study for my book *Bailey, Bach and Verbeia Flower Essences for Animals*, a pattern began to emerge. A reoccurrence that could not be classed as a coincidence was the number of animals that 'mirrored' the feelings of their owner to the exact same degree that they both needed to take the exact same flower essence combination. Our animals are very sensitive beings and just like a sponge will take on our own emotional baggage. They are so connected to us that on an energy level, they will mirror exactly what we are feeling.

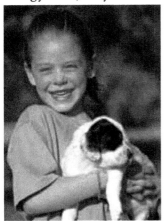

When I work with flower essences I like to connect to the energy of the animal. I ideally use some of the animal's fur (which is known as a witness), as this helps me to connect to their energy. Using a photograph, I can connect visually and also energetically. I try to have no preconceived ideas of what I think is going on, but let the animal speak to me via their energy. Using a pendulum, I dowse over each flower essence asking the question, 'Is this the essence that (name of animal) needs at this exact moment in time?' By asking this question, I can select the precise essence that is needed. If I use a question that is not so exact, there will often be a larger selection of flower essences chosen. The reason being that the animal may well require all of them, but not at this exact moment in time. It is here that the flower essences start to talk to me. They share their story of how the animal is feeling. Through the properties of the essences, I can understand the animal and comprehend why they are behaving in a certain way.

Also, the choice of essences will often 'reflect' the exact emotional problems of their owners. I have asked myself the question: why? What are the advantages for the animal? Every animal has a survival code; survival is engrained in their very being. Why would they become entrenched in our emotional problems? What are the advantages for them? Or at the simplest level, is it not the greatest gift of empathy that our animals can show us by reflecting the issues that we as owners need to address?

As I have said before, everything is energy; the lowest feelings vibrate at the lowest levels. When we are in the energy of a negative or unhappy person, you can immediately feel their energy bringing you down. Our animals easily and completely resonate with our negative feelings. Animals are wonderful teachers; as I get older and have spent time with lots of different animals, I have realised that they teach us in the most non-confrontational way; they quietly lead us to the correct answer, we just must listen with our heart. When the flower essences chosen are a mirror of the owner, I strongly recommend that the owner takes the remedy, too. We have a responsibility to ourselves and to our animals. The point being that our animals are showing us what we need to sort in ourselves. If it takes your animal to get you to sort out 'you', then there is no greater kindness.

When you work with energies, you realise that there is this whole invisible world that is full of magic. You realise that we communicate with our feelings, even though we are unaware of this fact. The smile, the laughter, praise and love vibrate at the highest level. These feelings are contagious and cascade like a stone dropped into a pond, enveloping everything in its path. This energy is beautiful, light and pure. If it were a song it would be musically brilliant as it would raise our emotions so that we would feel good. I like to imagine that flower essences are musical notes, the reason being that each one vibrates with their own unique energy to raise our animal's feelings.

Through my many years of using flower essences with animals and children, I have found that there is a perfect remedy 'melody' which works perfectly with the emotional problems that are being exhibited. If I tweak or tinker with any of the remedy, it stops working and almost immediately the owner or parent will say, 'What have you done to this remedy? It is different.' I will ask, 'How so?' The answer can be 'my animal is not responding how he usually does' or 'my daughter always sings when she takes the remedy and is not now'. Why do I need to tinker and tweak? It is my ingrained training, because Dr Bach described the essences as working on emotional layers, just like peeling an onion, and that is what initially I would do. I would think to myself: Where is the next layer of emotions? But in hindsight it was my ego wanting to change the perfect 'melody' as this was something I had been taught to do. As often as I changed the remedy, I always had to go back to the perfect 'melody'.

Some of my clients have been on the exact same remedy for three or more years. I started to listen to the animals and realised that they were teaching me to be patient, and to understand that we each individually have a 'unique' song that is specific to us. Just like our DNA there is our own 'specific' remedy that feeds our soul and allows us to be the person or animal we are meant to be. It allows us to connect to our deepest souls' desires and plays at the perfect vibration; it is magical. When I started my research, this was not something that I expected or even looked for, I thought I understood how flower essences work. I really did. Like everything in life, if we take the time to listen, and let go of our 'ego', a multitude of things can happen.

The Acupunture Set

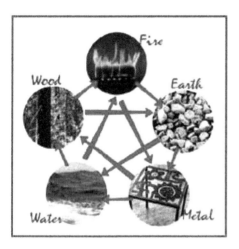

The Bailey Flower Essences are very unique as they have developed a range that work with the five elements. Although originally called the Acupuncture Set, the five-element flower essences set has been specially formulated for easy selection by any practitioner who uses meridians in their practice. It is based on the five-elements principles, and so can be used by anyone with a basic knowledge of the five elements.

Control and Creation Cycle

Let me explain the elements. I will try to keep this really simple, as the Chinese Five Elements are a huge topic in their own right. As we move through life, situations and experiences we can become each element. The five element cycle is fluid and not static; to be in balance each element needs to support the other elements. All five elements are equally important and should ideally be in balance, even though they are constantly being challenged. All materials are made from a single or combination of the five elements since these are the fundamental components of life. If the 'Water' element is blocked, then it would not be able to feed the 'Wood' element and this would have a knock-on effect of the 'Wood' element not being able to feed the 'Fire' element and so it goes. Your animal can also be defined as having specific personality traits of each element which can be in excess or in deficit.

The Water Animal

Have flowing movement like water with a glossy coat and tail. They have eyes to die for. Strong, dense, lean physique, sculptured face, high forehead, long narrow head, deep set eyes, broader at hips, long sensitive legs. They are highly sensitive, especially to noise.

Water Deficient

When Water is deficient, the presenting qualities might include fearfulness, despondency, inability to stick to anything, poor memory, lack of will power, premature aging, loss of libido, feelings of anxiety.

Water Excess

When Water is in excess, the presenting qualities might include recklessness, over-ambition, over-dominance, excessive sexual desire, jealousy, holding a grudge. Lack of judgement in people or other animals.

The Wood Animal

Can sometimes look stiff or wooden even though they can move quickly, they have a muscular lean square physique, thick coarse coat and feel firm to touch. They like a challenge and hate to be blocked.

Wood Deficient

When Wood is deficient, the presenting qualities may include lack of control, inability to plan, poor judgement, poor co-ordination, no life/ soul purpose and depression.

Wood Excess

When Wood is in excess, the presenting qualities may include over-controlling and they may overdo it. They feel stuck and inflexible, and lash out in frustration.

The Fire Animal

Has the 'electric' personality that turns heads. They stride out gracefully with elegance. Their willowy long neck, limbs and fine thin coat stand out. They feel soft and velvety to touch. They like excitement but once their fire has burnt out they become despondent.

Fire Deficient
When Fire is deficient, the presenting qualities might include lack of joy, inability to speak, cold extremities, apathy, depression, exhaustion, inability to love, hatred, despondency, relying on others for a sense of identity.

Fire Excess
When Fire is in excess, the presenting qualities might include compulsiveness, desire for permanent joy, aggression, impatience, impulsiveness, going over the top, going too far, frenzy and over-agitation.

The Earth Animal

Has round, well-muscled, broad physique with an overriding tendency to be fat. They move rhythmically yet heavily. They often have rather scruffy coats and feel fleshy to touch. They like routine, stability and don't appreciate change.

Earth Deficient
When Earth is deficient, the presenting qualities might include loss of appetite, lack of metal clarity, over-thinking, worrying, needy, clingy, unsympathetic, easily led, lethargic, ungrounded, self-centred.

Earth Excess
When Earth is in excess, the presenting qualities might include being over protective of others, smothering, overly sympathetic, overly responsible, obsessive, obstinate, stubborn, seeking sympathy, over-eating.

The Metal Animal

Look slightly angular with delicate features; they have small bones, compact muscles, with a coat that has a tendency to be dry and brittle. They like structure and can often appear inflexible like metal.

Metal Deficient
When Metal is deficient, the presenting qualities may include being unable to relate to others, loss of structure, feeling disconnected, melancholy, suffering with prolonged grief.

Metal Excess
When Metal is in excess, the presenting qualities may include rigid thinking, and a person may be unreceptive to new ideas, controlled and controlling, overly analytical, overly ambitious, unyielding. Rigid and snappish if needs for order and creativeness are not met.

Using The Five Element Set With Animals

It is not going to be easy to identify that your animal is deficient or in excess of a specific element and also exactly which element will apply to your animal at a specific time. I have devised a questionnaire which will help you to find out which element your animal is in the first instance.

Interpreting the Results
Read the question for each element and only answer 'yes' to the answer that applies. When answering, think about your animal and not what the species would do in that situation. For example, although a cat would run from something scary, how does your cat cope with that situation? They may still run away but are they stubborn? Frenzied? Despondent? The element with the highest number will be your animal's dominant element and will indicate to you how they see the world. By understanding your animal's element, you will be able to understand their thought process and therefore understand what drives them daily and also their strengths and weakness. You will be able to support their element with the acupuncture set so they will always be in balance. To find if your animal is deficient or in excess then you will

need to refer to the descriptions in this book. Your animal can also be a combination of two or more elements; in this case, think of how they cope in varying settings to work out the dominant element. Use your initiative and feel the element that is being expressed. The five elements are not set in stone and are always constantly changing just like your animal is. Try to feel what your animal is expressing to you and be open with your mind.

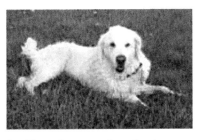

Water Element

1. Is it trusting by nature?
2. Prefers to be in the background of activity?
3. Can it be fussy or demanding?
4. Can be withdrawn or depressed?
5. Does it ever give the impression of being 'miles away'?
6. Stubborn or apathetic?
7. Dislikes being rushed?
8. Can harbour deep fears?
9. Takes a while to warm up to new people?
10. Can be easily overwhelmed by noise?

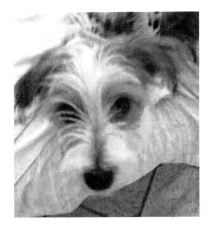

Wood Element

1. Always on the go?
2. Can lash out?
3. Does not like being confined?
4. Does it habitually have angry outbursts?
5. Pushes the boundaries to test limits?
6. Is it often impatient?
7. Enjoys being the leader?
8. Does it enjoy a challenge?
9. Easily bored?
10. Finds it difficult to keep still?

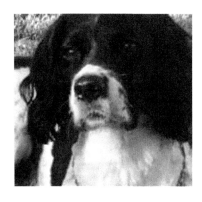

Fire Element

1. Loves to be the centre of attention?
2. Does this animal get panicky?
3. Can be impulsive and over-stimulated?
4. Can it get over-exuberant?
5. Enjoys entertaining others?
6. Is it shy?
7. Friendly and enthusiastic?
8. Can turn on a dime?
9. Charismatic?
10. Needs constant attention?

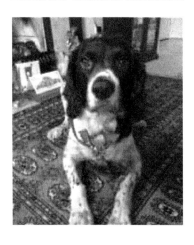

Earth Element

1. Loves being in a group setting (herd/pack)?
2. Does it get overly concerned or worry about others?
3. Outgoing but does not want to be the centre of attention?
4. Is it emotionally needy?
5. Good at making friends?
6. Does it respond well to changes in routine?
7. Attached to their owner?
8. Tendency to put on weight?
9. Home orientated?
10. Does not like conflict within the home?

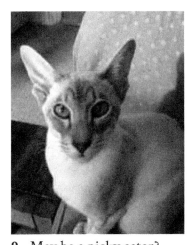

Metal Element

1. Prefers routine?
2. Sweet & gentle but also stubborn?
3. Does it respect boundaries of others?
4. Is it sensitive about its personal space?
5. Will follow the rules?
6. Can it seem aloof?
7. Sensitive to the environment?
8. Sensitive to the owner's emotions?
9. May be a picky eater?
10. Unbending when their mind is made up?

Case Study 3

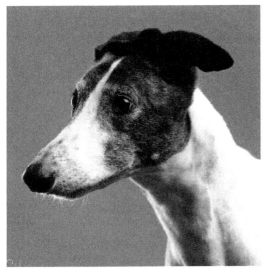

Paddy is a greyhound that I have been working with for a few years. He is a dog who was highly reactive to other dogs and hated cats. He did not cope well when there were lots of people and dogs around. He was also food aggressive and had bitten other dogs, even those that he knew well. He would become fixated with other dogs, showing his teeth in an antisocial fashion.

The first thing that I needed to treat was his aggression, which I immediately saw as 'fear aggression'. When he had exhausted all attempts to avoid an aggressive encounter, he had learnt that by biting other dogs, this had the desired result to ward other dogs away. If he got in first with his bout of aggression, he was always rewarded with the other dog moving out of his space. The fears he had were caused by a lack of socialisation when he was a puppy, and his food aggression was caused by a cat stealing his food when he was a puppy. He had learnt to guard his food at all costs and to do this he needed to be aggressive if there were other dogs around.

The first thing I needed to do was to treat his fear issues combined with his lack of control in lashing out. So I chose the following Bailey essences.

Buttercup – To bring the sunshine back into his life.

Mahonia – Which allowed him to move forward.

Sea Campion – To help him deal with the early separation from his mother.

Ragwort – To break his fixation with other dogs and cats.

The result after a few months was that Paddy firstly became less food aggressive with the amazing result that he did not actually care much for the brand of dog food, yet had been guarding it and eating it in the fear that someone would steal it. The Bailey essences allowed Paddy to be less fearful when he was out with other dogs, so he was able to learn that when a dog came into his space it was okay. He became more social and his owner was not stressed that he was going to bite another dog. Paddy picked up on the new calmer energy of his owner, which resulted in a quieter Paddy. He was also fed on a raw food diet, so he had no additives, which could also affect his behaviour.

One of the many messages from his owner:

'Paddy's remedy arrived yesterday. Love the green bottle! He is eating much slower and much less aggressive around food which is great. He has decided that if he doesn't like something he doesn't have to eat it. Before you could almost see him holding his nose and forcing himself to eat it because it was food. We still supervise feeding more to make sure that Neva eats hers. Will keep you posted on his progress. Cx'

I still treat Paddy and he has grown in to a confident older dog, who is now not so reactive to other dogs and has an inner calmness and is at peace.

Grief and Bailey, Bach qnd Verbeia Flower Essences

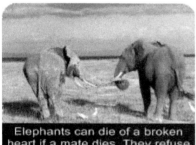

Elephants can die of a broken heart if a mate dies. They refuse to eat and will lay down, shedding tears until they starve to death.

I lost my father some years ago after he had suffered from a long illness. For the last 15 months of his life my father was in a place where he had lost the use of his legs, he had lost his independence and he had definitely lost the will to live. As the 15 months unfolded there were so many emotional ups and downs. At no point could I relax and there was no time where I could truly think. My mind was fogged, my decisions were flawed, but most of all I experienced deep anxiety. It was like living in a space that was not connected to this world, yet at the same time I needed to function on a daily basis. Grief is different for everyone; my twin sister was totally devastated, crying every day, unable to get out of bed. Yet I managed to hold down my job, change to a new job and to find a place within myself that allowed me to function on a day-to-day basis. However the news of my father's death hit me like a train wreck.

Charles Darwin wrote a book in 1872 called 'The Expression of Emotion in Man and Animals'. He concluded that animals clearly felt emotions, given the similarity between human and animal behaviour. He wrote 'The young and the old of widely different races, both with man and animals, express the same state of mind by the same movements'. Scientists are still researching, studying, compiling evidence to support/discredit Darwin's original theories. Yet when you look at your dog when you return from work, you can just see the joy and happiness in their face. You can see how they feel when they go to the vet; you can see their disappointment when they don't get their walk, the excitement when they get their favourite toy. However, we are still studying them, trying to prove that we are the higher race. Darwin was a very clever man and in honesty it does not take a lot of brain power to see that our animals truly do have emotions. We certainly do not have a monopoly on grief. They feel everything that we feel: disappointment, love, grief, fear and even shame. I have seen my own two dogs who on every single occasion run down stairs each morning to be let out; but on the days they have been mischievous during the night, they hold back until I have gone into the kitchen to see the mounds of tissues scattered all over the floor.

For some reason we expect our animals to be immune to grief; it is not something that is intentional or misplaced, it is because we miss the signs. They may not cry like we do but when you observe them, there are clear indications of grief; looking melancholy, refusing to eat, pacing the floor, lack of interest, howling and barking. When you think about it from their point of view, their owner has taken their poor companion to the vet; they wait patiently for your return and in you come, empty-handed. We don't explain why we are tearful or where their friend is (maybe some of you do); they in turn spend days looking for their companion while we openly grieve. We don't mean to be so insensitive, it is just human nature.

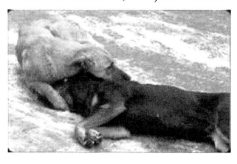

Treat them as you would with anyone who has lost a loved one. Being of Irish descent, I returned to Ireland for my dad's funeral. The custom is that they are buried in three days after their death and they are brought home in an open coffin. I and my husband argued all of the way from the airport about seeing my father dead in the coffin. As I entered my home and saw my grieving family sitting around his coffin, I gulped in a state of shock. I, too, was seated with my family as a procession of people entered the house shaking each one of our hands and saying 'sorry for your loss'. They then stood next to his coffin and reflected on their own thoughts. My husband and my 21- and 18-year-old sons ushered people into the room as streams of people came to pay their respects. Over the next few hours something unexpected happened, having my dead father in the living room became normal; it was not scary, it was almost like he was still part of the family. It helped my sons to understand death. My father stayed overnight and one of us slept in the room with him so he would not be alone. What I dreaded most was seeing my father in a coffin, but in honesty it just felt so natural. It got me thinking about how unnaturally we treat death in relation to our animals. After my own experience I truly feel that it's **so** important that your animal can see the dead body of their companion. By doing this they are more able to come to terms with what has happened to their companion.

'When someone you love becomes a memory, the memory becomes a treasure.'
(Unknown)
'All the darkness in the world cannot extinguish the light of a single candle.'
(Saint Francis of Assisi)

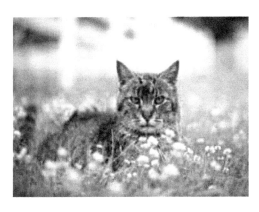

Bailey, Bach and Verbeia Flower Essences for Grief

Trailing St John's Wort – Takes the sting out of the situation and reduces the emotional tension and desperation that are part of your animal's grieving process.

Yorkshire Fog – Encourages shedding of tears and symbolically washes away the anguish that naturally occurs at such times.

Dog Rose – Offers loving comfort support when your animal is totally bereft.

Sheep's Sorrel – Helps your animal to let go of resentment and foreboding feelings that 'it always happens to them'.

Star of Bethlehem – Is the essence for shock and grief and will help your animal to grieve.

Honeysuckle – Will help your animal to move forward and to accept the future by letting go of the pain of the past.

Soft Rush – Offers a nurturing loving hug when all feels lost.

In precisely the same way you would treat your animal, take the Bailey, Bach and Verbeia essences to help heal your own grief. Animals often 'mirror' our own emotional feelings, so don't be surprised if the essences you need are exactly the same as your animals.

Take two drops from your chosen essence and mix it with 30mls of spring water in a treatment bottle. Shake vigorously and give four drops from this bottle to your animal four times a day.

'If having a soul means being able to feel love and loyalty and gratitude, then animals are better off than a lot of humans.' (James Herriot)

Case Study 4

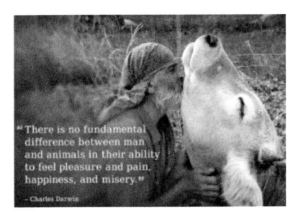

"There is no fundamental difference between man and animals in their ability to feel pleasure and pain, happiness, and misery."

- Charles Darwin

This is the second time I am asked to treat Otis and it is because he sadly loses two of the dogs from his pack very suddenly and is now an only dog. He is very stressed and starts damaging the house and furniture. He also starts urinating in his home.

Otis is going through a difficult time of change, grief, perhaps even loneliness. The essences that I have chosen will help Otis to move forward, so he can feel safe and secure and in time be happy again.

Yorkshire Fog will enable Otis to open up to the pain of grief. Accepting hurt or grief is part of the healing process for him. It is a definite fact that animals grieve and need to process the loss of another animal or person. It is often very difficult for owners of animals to know whether their animal is grieving as they don't wail or shed tears as a human would. Yorkshire Fog will help Otis to be open to grief, so he can express it more honestly.

Leopardsbane is the essence for animals that are living on a knife-edge and seeing this in Otis can be very distressing. The negative aspect of the Leopardsbane characteristic is that it can lead to serious depression and even to suicidal thoughts. Because of the powerful emotions generated in such states, there is often a real problem with addiction to the feelings of negativity. Animals in this state are often shut down as they are trapped in in their own suffering. Leopardsbane is useful in two ways: first, in lessening the attachment to emotional extremes; second, in allowing the perceptions to broaden.

I think that we both can agree that Otis is grieving as he has lost two of his beloved pack members within a very short time.

The essences chosen are an interesting combination and they will work by raising Otis's vibrations, which have been influenced by his grief. They start to vibrate at a lower frequency and the impact of this affects Otis's emotional wellbeing. The flower essences energy is at a higher frequency and when Otis takes it his frequency will be influenced by the energy too; eventually he will oscillate at the same frequency as the flower essences. The point is that giving him the whole bottle will be equivalent to giving him four drops. It is the frequency of the doses and not the quantity. (Plus it only works if he has it regularly.)

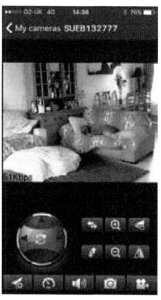

Flower essences take from 24 hours to a couple of weeks to show change. The essence needs to be kept in the fridge. Let me know how you get on. There is much love from me too on the way to you both.

With love,
Caroline xx

The result was that the Bailey Flower Essences started to work very quickly. His owner purchased a camera so that she could watch him while she was at work. She took a picture of him totally chilled out on his sofa. He stopped urinating and he eventually became very playful and very happy with being an only dog.

Mental Health Issues

We can be forgiven for thinking that mental health issues are only obvious in the human race. Having lost my brother and nephew to suicide, I have an understanding of what it is like to live with two young men with severe mental health issues. When was the tipping point so great that they both took their own lives? I will never truly know, but what I do know is that life was too painful; in the end death was the only option. To lose two young men had a huge impact on my family; there have been many years filled with grief and sadness, but it has allowed me to have empathy, understanding, and it has given me the desire to study this complex subject. There is a lot of truth in the saying that 'you have to walk the walk, to talk the talk'. Mental health issues in young people are at an all-time high; appointments with psychiatrists are taking up to nine months, which is leaving vulnerable people without the necessary help that they need. The issue is very close to my heart. If we cannot understand the mental health issues of our children, how are we going to understand those in our animals?

Now there is so much more evidence that some of animals in our lives are in a constant state of stress. They frequently suffer with allergies, skin conditions, anxiety and fear. I have treated many animals with symptoms of stress; and when I take a look at the problem at a deeper level, there is always a point in their lives where something has happened and often a point when something is missing, which does not give them the necessary tools to deal with day-to-day life. What happens if this stress is never addressed and the animal is constantly being pushed into a state of anxiety? In exactly the same way as humans, they start to exhibit behaviours that serve no purpose other than to relieve their stress.

Picture the patient rocking backwards and forwards in a mental institute; the rocking is rhythmic and often caresses their mind to help reduce their spiralling state of anxiety. Animals, too, are showing more and more similar behaviours, which in the animal world is termed 'stereotypical behaviour'. These behaviours can be seen in the horse weaving in the stable, the cat licking its leg until it bleeds, the horse licking the stable walls and the stallion biting his flank even when it is already a gapping open wound. These are examples of animals I have worked with; some of them I could help, with amazing results; but it was the ones that I could not help that made me ask why. What pushes an animal to the place of no return? It is often caused by a lack of understanding of what the animal needs, and then the behaviour becomes so engrained that it becomes impossible to fix. Even when you take all of the stress away, the animal is unable to change.

A professor of neurosurgery in California, Phil Weinstein, has said that animals feel anxiety similar to humans because the structure of their brain involved in the responses is not that different to ours. Therefore, this being the case, there comes the possibility of a mental breakdown. Learning about fear is often triggered using the 'flight and fight' response. It is the body's primitive, automatic, inborn response that prepares the body to 'fight' or 'flee' from actual or perceived attack, harm or threat to protect their survival. When activated, everything becomes a possible treat or danger. This response is triggered across all species and was an important tool to protect them from the possible threats of the sabre-toothed tiger.

Alas, there are no tigers today, and yet the 'flight and fight' response is continually being triggered by perceived fears that our animals are unable to process. They are often in a situation where they are unable to flee, as these perceived fears can often take place in the home, such as the postman posting the letters through the letter box while the owner is at work. They cannot fight either, yet their fears are real. Each time the response is triggered it releases toxic hormones into their body, which would have been dissipated naturally if the animal was allowed to flee and fight. There are no sabre-toothed tigers, yet the animal's body is continually in a state of anxiety. The hormones are continually being triggered, causing an array of health problems. Issues such as immune disorders, skin problems, and more importantly, emotional or psychological symptoms are manifesting as anxiety, depression, sadness or fear. Many anxieties will directly manifest in the physical body, taking the form of excessive licking, weaving and feather-plucking.

If the animal's mother was very fearful and not socialised properly, she would not have been able to teach her baby with confidence and it is often the case that this fear is passed on to her young. When you combine the 'flight and fight response' with faulty genetics you have a higher possibility that the animal will find it difficult and sometimes impossible to cope under stressful situations.

Early socialisation is the most important gift you can offer your animal to help them to understand that the world is not full of tigers. Try to see things from your animal's point of view by recognising stressful situations. How is it making them feel? Flower essences can make a huge difference in helping your animal emotionally to cope with anxiety and fear. I have worked with animals that have been transformed from a quivering wreck into having a more carefree attitude to life. You have to make sure that you remove the triggers that are causing the stress, so that the flower essences can work fully. If you cannot remove the stress triggers then you will need to work with your animal, so that you can socialise them to the situation or object. The flower essences support the animals while they learn to deal with their fears, they will relieve the anxieties, so life is not a scary place.

So what about the animals that I couldn't save? As it is the law in the UK to work with a vet, if you are to treat an animal that is not your own, I was able to share my understandings and assessment of these situations. The vet is responsible for the health and welfare of the animal and also is able to offer a greater insight into the situation. Recognising that a client may be beyond your capabilities is at the heart of what makes a good Animal Holistic Practitioner. The ones I could not save received intensive veterinary and behavioural treatment to help them to let go of their anxieties.

Bailey, Bach and Verbeia Flower Essences aor Fear

Betony is for unrecognisable fears, fears that can make us feel unloved, unwanted or unworthy. Betony helps us to see that such fears are groundless by shedding light in the dark places of the mind.

Mahonia helps to free us from the fear of our own inner power. Such fear usually arises from seeing the immense damage that can be caused by fanatical people. Yet those who fear their own power are those who are the most trustworthy, the least likely to misuse that personal power.

Greater Celandine is for those who fear their spiritual nature. Many of us have put up, however unwittingly, a mental block between ourselves and the source of our existence. Often this is because the logical mind, once more, does not want to accept dimensions of reality that it cannot understand, and over which it has no control. This fear of the non-physical can produce many different problems.

Mimulus is the essence for known fears such as those of the postman, vet or other animals etc.

Aspen is the essence for fears of the unknown, such as those that cause your animal to be afraid when there is no reason as to why they are in a state of fear.

Rock Rose is the most powerful essence for animals who are completely so shaken by fear that they cannot move.

Fylfot will allow your animal to feel safe and secure when faced with a fearful situation.

Early Abrupt Weaning

Christmas is the time of year when humans are giving and inclined to purchase cute kittens and puppies as gifts for their family. The initial union is filled with much optimism and happiness; but after a few days, the reality of looking after a kitten or puppy starts to become apparent. The strain on the family from sleepless nights, or the smell of wee and poo, causes the owners to justify their behaviour of shouting and hitting their baby animal for all of the wrongdoings that have occurred. Next come the excuses as to why they cannot keep the baby animal, how the animal has caused them so much stress. We have barely reached New Year's Eve and the baby animal is now coming to terms with a new home in a Rescue Centre.

Let us wind back to the beginning of this baby animal's life, nestled in the bosom of their mother with their siblings keeping them warm. Life is very simple, with nothing more to do than eat and sleep. In the wild, feral kittens would stay with their mother for up to eight months and puppies, if allowed to follow their wolf relations, would stay with their mother for up to 18 months. Yet we humans have a magical number of eight weeks. In reality, it makes sense to the breeder as the babies are growing rapidly, therefore eating more; their hearing and eyesight is developed and they are becoming more aware of the big wide world around them. Unfortunately, in some baby animals, especially those younger than eight weeks, being taken from their mother so early can cause a catalogue of behavioural problems. Hence, taking us back to the original opening paragraph, our lack of animal understanding, and early abrupt weaning can have catastrophic possibilities for the baby animal.

The simplest way to describe why behavioural problems would manifest is to look at it from another point of view. For example: a young child taken from a family and forced to live in the wild, with wolves, has not learnt the basics of how to be 'human' from their mother or siblings. There have been documented cases of feral children in the past, which showed that they lacked basic human skills such as how to use a toilet, how to stand up straight. The biggest revelation is their complete lack of interest in any human activity. They are disconnected with the human world around them. We are in essence doing the same to our animals, by taking them from their mother at such a young age and expecting them to understand the laws of the human world, even though they have barely learnt the laws of their own animal kingdom. If a dog does not learn that he is a dog and how to communicate with dogs, there will be a blurred line of an animal being a dog, but thinking they are human as they have been taken away from their mother far too young. We then expect them to play nicely with the dogs in the park, but in reality, they have not learnt the skills and dog language to do so. They become fearful of other dogs, and this fear often turns into an outburst of barking and biting, from which then they are then labelled aggressive. Animals who have been taken from their mothers often feel that the world is scary; cats will spend a lot of their life hiding and dogs will often find it difficult to relate to other dogs.

It needs to be understood that for animals that suffer from early abrupt weaning, a lot of their problems are due to them feeling fearful and insecure. They find new experiences scary as they do not have the communication or social skills to deal with them. They like routine and can be unpredictable when pushed outside their comfort zone. Re-socialising them to new practices will take time, so move slowly and allow them to show you the pace that you both need to work with. Flower essences can play a big part in helping them to adjust.

Bailey, Bach and Verbeia to the Rescue

Bailey essences can be used to support rescue animals. We live in a world where all and sundry seems to think that everything is disposable; our clothes, our food and even our animals. Some of us humans breed animals for financial gain, although I believe that comment would be disputed by the majority. They gloss over the fact that rescue centres around the world are bursting at the seams with animals that are waiting to be placed in a new home. The sad fact is that it is about the money and there is no way that they can know how the lives will turn out.

There are many reasons why animals end up at a shelter, the main one being that the animal is no longer wanted. There are numerous excuses as to the reason why they cannot keep their pet. Here in the UK, a person brought a dog into a rescue centre because he did not match her curtains! There are, of course, very genuine heartfelt reasons why animals go to a shelter; and these cannot be underestimated as to the impact on the owner and animal. Below is a selection of reasons that have often been used.

- He is too old
- He is too young
- He is too expensive to keep
- He is too hard to handle
- He has wrecked my home
- He barks all day and night
- I am moving home and I cannot take him with me
- I have just got divorced and cannot keep him
- My children are allergic to him
- I cannot afford the vet bills

- He pooped in my kitchen
- He peed on my bed
- I am too old to keep my dog
- I am too young to have a dog

If you look at the above individually or collectively, the emotional feelings of the animal will be a different combination of different feelings: fear, grief, loss, shock, change, uncertainty, sadness, despair and a sense of being heartbroken. Each animal will react differently to the new situation that they have been thrust into. The animal will either draw on a past experience as a coping mechanism, or the whole situation will be so overwhelming that they will withdraw into the furthest corner of the kennel/cage.

By addressing each animal as an individual with Bailey, Bach and Verbeia essences, you will be able to get to the heart of the emotional problem. It will make it easier for the animal to be re-homed and will ultimately raise the optimism of the animal. There is of course the more difficult subject of abuse, where the animal has experienced cruelty from the hands of a human. Here the emotional wounds are deeper and more ingrained into the very soul of the animal. Bailey, Bach and Verbeia essences have an important part to play here also, as they are able to work layer by emotional layer, to get to the true inner core of the animal. I have worked with horses, where their lifeless eyes and demeanour meant they had given up on the human race and themselves. By combining a selection of flower essences and giving it to them over a few weeks, it was amazing to see their trust and friendship start to shine through, to eventually be spirited and carefree with the other animals and people.

Lesser Stitchwort helps us disentangle ourselves from our difficulties. It can then act as a guiding star, showing us clearly the path ahead that we need to be following.

Butterbur is for those who have had their self-esteem damaged from an early age. They may well feel inadequate because of adverse comments from parents and teachers early in their lives. They may have become convinced that in some way, they are unworthy. Butterbur liberates and opens the way for the discovery of innate strengths and wisdom.

Moss is for those who fear the dark spaces within their being. They do not recognise their innate goodness, surrounded as it may be by a mass of negative conditioning. Moss helps us to see that it is only our fears that we are really frightened of.

Walnut will support change and will allow your animal to adapt to any new situation that comes their way.

Winberry will help your animal to move forward in a complete and helpful way.

Fear of Fireworks

Fireworks are being used more and more as a way for us to celebrate; they are now commonplace at birthday parties, Christmas celebrations and New Year's celebrations. While we may enjoy the brightly coloured flashes and loud sounds, unfortunately most of our pets don't appreciate the noise with quite the same enthusiasm. They have extra sensitive hearing and can find this time of year extremely stressful, even traumatic.

Some animals cope with fireworks and other loud noises fine, but a lot of the animals I have treated are terrified. Your pet will behave in the way its species would behave if in the wild... horses will run, cats usually like to climb up high, dogs like to bark and howl. Respect them for their 'coping' mechanisms. Knowing your pet and how they react is key to having a happy well-balanced pet during the fireworks celebration.

Signs of stress are:
- Shaking
- Excessive grooming
- Barking
- Marking the home
- Running away
- Soiling
- Being over-excited
- Running in circles
- Scratching at the furniture excessively
- Drooling

Having a plan as to how you are going to protect your animal from the loud noises and flashes will offer the best support for your animal.

If it is possible, try to obtain a recording or video of fireworks. Start playing it on the lowest sound level; this is called desensitisation, which is a process whereby you introduce your animal to the sound of the fireworks. To desensitise your animal, watch for the reaction of your animal to the sound, and turn it off immediately if you notice that your animal is stressed. Gradually, over a few weeks, increase the sound level and frequency of the recording or video. Do not rush the process as you will over-stress your animal; always be guided by them. It is good to distract them with a game or a treat.

Here are some simple tips to help your animals get through the next couple of months:

- Start giving Bailey, Bach and Verbeia Flower Essences about seven days before the fireworks celebration.
- Keep your pets indoors and provide them with a den where they can feel safe.
- Turn the TV up or play music. Classical music is by far the most soothing and can camouflage the outside sounds. Close the curtains. Bring rabbits and guinea pigs in from outside and place them in a safe place. Give them extra bedding to burrow in.
- Make sure doors and windows are securely shut, this is very important as it ensures your animal will not run off. Make sure your animal has been micro-chipped or at the very least name-tagged.
- Try not to reinforce fearful behaviour when they are anxious; animals are very sensitive and can pick up on our own anxiety. If you treat your animal like a human baby smothering them with cuddles, embraces and nuzzles when they are scared, you are reinforcing their fearful behaviour, which makes them feel worse.
- Allow them to hide in a bolthole, if needed. This is a natural response to something that they would fear. Don't coax your cat out of their hiding place. They will emerge in their own time.
- Distract them with a game of some kind, new toys or chews so they are not focused on the sound of the fireworks.
- Walk your dog in the daylight and make sure that they go to the toilet before and after the fireworks. Supply a litter tray for your cat.

If you really must get fireworks:
• Do not let fireworks off near your pet.
• Keep fireworks as far away from the home as possible.
• Buy silent fireworks – yes! They do exist.
• Buy handheld cascade fireworks.
• Go to a local display.

It is very important to check your bonfires before starting them as small animals, particularly hedgehogs, like to seek refuge in leaves as they tend to hibernate.

We as owners have a huge responsibility to provide a safe and stress-free environment for our animals. We have a duty where possible to ensure that our animals from an early age have been socialised to as many experiences as possible during their day-to-day lives.

Autism

As with children, here in the UK, there has been a big increase in the number of dogs with autism. I have been very privileged to be able to offer my flower essence skills to a study where owners of dogs with autism can share their experiences. It is believed that over-vaccinating of our dogs is the 'trigger', which is highly suspected to be the same cause in children, too. The difference is that our children are only usually vaccinated once, to certain viruses, whereas dogs are vaccinated 'yearly' for the same diseases! It is a very basic biology fact that once vaccinated, the immunity of your dog should last for a lifetime.

Vaccination is a very controversial subject, as most of us have an annual holiday; we must abide by the conditions of the boarding kennels. Your dog must have had all their vaccinations and these must be up-to-date. So off we go to have another set of vaccinations done for diseases that 'Fido' is already immune to!

Signs Of Autism In Dogs

How can you recognise that your dog has autism? They behave in the same way as children with autism do. They find it very difficult to make eye contact with their owner, they dislike change, they are stressed by big crowds and they are highly sensitive to their surroundings. They are extremely difficult to control and can be very unpredictable. They find learning new things to be very difficult.

Palliatve Care

When you are faced with the impending death of your animal it is here that the Bailey, Bach and Verbeia essences can play a huge part in helping your animal to pass peacefully to the other side. Palliative care is often coupled with hospice care, which allows a pet owner to provide comfort care for a dying animal, usually in the home and with the assistance of a veterinarian or veterinary nurse. The most important aspect of palliative care is to keep your animal as pain free as possible. The medication used is as follows: nonsteroidal anti-inflammatory drugs (e.g., carprofen, meloxicam). In more severe episodes of pain then opioids can be used. (e.g. morphine, tramadol). It is very important to recognise the signs of pain within your animal. Animals can suffer from both acute pain and chronic pain. Acute pain is much easier to see; your animal will likely show obvious signs of being uncomfortable and may make noises, not lie on a certain part of the body and perhaps lick at an area. Chronic pain can be a little harder to observe. Changes in your animal's behaviour, such as incontinence or increased anxiety, can also signal that they are in pain.

Effective palliative care requires the expertise of a veterinarian, preferably one with special training and interest in hospice and palliative care. All vets are trained to treat pain and can help you come up with a careful plan. It is up to you to observe and report physical and behavioural changes in your animal to the veterinarian. You are your animal's eyes to the world and also their voice, so please be very vigilant in how you assess your animal's pain.

The goal is not to prolong suffering. In fact, the goal is to prevent suffering and to allow your animal to live as long as possible, until death occurs or euthanasia is necessary. To convert your home into an animal hospice you just need to make it animal friendly and easy to use. Have a safe comfy place with lots of soft blankets. Make sure it is quiet and is not in a place where lots of people walk through. Raise their food and water bowl so that they are easier to use. Make sure they have access to the outside should they need to go to the toilet.

I have created some special exercises which will help you through this very sad time.

MAGICAL MOMENTS

You will need a pen and note pad
Find a quiet space with your animal and share all of the magical moments you have had together. Speak from the heart and not with suddenness but with love
Take a deep breath and write down these moments. They are not to make you feel sad but to help you to understand that death comes to all of us. The biggest gift you can give to your animal is to fill their last days with happy energy. However difficult this may be for you, your animal will be very sensitive to how you are feeling right now and the last thing you want to do is for them to feel sad for you.

FLOWER POWER

As soon as you make the very sad decision to have your animal put to sleep, both you and your animal will need Bailey flower support, so you can be emotionally strong for your animal and so that your animal is emotionally ready.

- Bistort
- Heath Bedstraw
- Single Snowdrop
- Yorkshire Fog
- Star of Bethlehem

Add two drops from the stock bottle, mix with spring water and give four drops four times a day.

GRATITUDE MEDITATION

Close your eyes and take three deep breaths; imagine you are with your animal in a beautiful green meadow. The sun is warm as you find a place to sit. Your animal comes and lies by your feet. You look into their eyes and they look into your eyes too. The deep feeling of love that you feel between each other is so powerful and consuming. Spend the next five minutes feeling gratitude for all the amazing things that your animal has given to you unconditionally and with much love in their heart.
Thank your animal and then open your eyes.

OUR SPECIAL PLACE

By creating a special imaginary place for your animal, it will allow you and your animal to connect on a deeper spiritual level. The place could be a meadow, a beach, a forest or any special place you can think of.

Sit, feel your feet comfortably on the floor and close your eyes. Remember a place in your life where you and your animal had been able to share some wonderful memories. Imagine, see, feel, this place in your mind and allow it to become a welcoming beautiful place for you to share with your animal. Make the 'Special Place' as comfortable as possible; you could add cushions, or throws. Invite your animal into this special place. Do they run in? Walk in? Are they timid or excited? Allow them to have a look around and invite them to come and sit next to you. Spend 10 – 15 minutes in this space. Have no expectations, just offer love.

Index